CHRONIC PAIN

PSYCHOSOCIAL FACTORS IN REHABILITATION

This volume is one of the series,
Rehabilitation Medicine Library,
Edited by John V. Basmajian

* Originally published as part of the Physical Medicine Library, edited by Sidney Licht.

Chronic Pain

Psychosocial Factors in Rehabilitation

Edited by *Ranjan*

R. Roy, ADV. DIP. S.W.

**School of Social Work
and Department of Psychiatry,
University of Manitoba, Winnipeg, Canada**

E. Tunks, M.D., F.R.C.P.(C.)

**Department of Psychiatry and Pain Clinic,
Chedoke-McMaster Hospital and
McMaster University School of Medicine,
Hamilton, Ontario, Canada**

WILLIAMS & WILKINS
Baltimore/London

Copyright ©, 1982
Williams & Wilkins
428 E. Preston Street
Baltimore, Md. 21202, U.S.A.

Made in the United States of America

Library of Congress Cataloging in Publication Data

Main entry under title:

Chronic pain.

(Rehabilitation medicine library)
Includes index.
1. Pain—Treatment.   2. Psychotherapy.   3. Pain—Psychological   aspects.
4. Pain—Social aspects. 5. Chronically ill—Rehabilitation. I. Roy, R. (Ranjan)
II. Tunks, E. (Eldon) III. Series. [DNLM: 1. Pain, Intractable—Psychology.
2. Pain, Intractable—Rehabilitation. WL 704 C5585]
RB127.C5   616′.0472   81-13101
ISBN 0-683-07394-X   AACR2

Composed and printed at the
Waverly Press, Inc.
Mt. Royal and Guilford Aves.
Baltimore, MD 21202, U.S.A.

Series Editor's Foreword

As the *Rehabilitation Medicine Library* enlarges, I am faced with the pleasant problem of avoiding phrases and words I have used to praise my editors and their new volumes. "Unique?" Certainly that adjective applies to this work which will stand as a landmark in rehabilitation. "Deeply involved and intelligent specialists?" No question about it: the editors have chosen some of the top minds in this field and have woven the text skillfully. They themselves are leading thinkers and practitioners in the field of chronic pain and rehabilitation and so their substantial contributions to the chapters add a special dimension.

Chronic pain today looms as an epidemic. An integrated approach to rehabilitation of those who are handicapped by it has emerged as a major function of many related professions. No group has more to offer than the multidisciplinary rehabilitation team.

In isolation, any one specialist becomes frustrated and impotent to manage both severe and moderate cases—and even mild cases. This book offers a substantial foundation for improved management of the whole range of musculoskeletal pain problems. In particular it offers the "lone-ranger" practitioner some guidelines to the most successful approach that I am aware of.

The restoration to more useful and productive lives of all patients with debilitating chronic pain problems seen in orthopaedic and general practice and in rehabilitation facilities is our ultimate aim. But first, all health professionals must know what is written in this book if the epidemic of chronic pain is to be brought under good control.

JOHN V. BASMAJIAN, M.D.

Preface

The idea for this book was conceived when one of us (R.R.) left McMaster to take up a position at another university. As is often the case, once removed from the situation, it seemed important to give shape to the experience of the long years of association with the Pain Clinic and its members. To this end, we began to conceptualize our theoretical and clinical approaches which culminated in the birth of this book. This book is the result of our collective experience as practising clinicians at the McMaster University Pain Clinic in Hamilton, Canada. We became acutely aware that we were essentially engaged in the rehabilitation process with our patients with chronic pain. Reconstitution of weakened defenses, restoration of lost roles and resumption of normal family life for our patients were and remain major objectives of treatment at the Pain Clinic. The biomedical model seemed singularly inadequate for helping this group of patients. In a curious way, as far as the pain patient is concerned, there is often no 'disease' to treat. On the other hand, psychological and social factors are universally recognized as significant contributors to the etiology and maintenance of chronic pain. Treatment strategies, therefore, have a strong psychosocial emphasis.

For that reason, we have attempted in this book a sociopsychological conceptualization of the pain problem, and it is our hope that the book will be of practical value for practitioners working with this most challenging group of patients. We consider ourselves very fortunate in that so many of our contributors, who are seminal thinkers in this field, agreed to make original contributions. Equally, we are proud of the fact that many of our associates at McMaster University consented to share their unique perspectives and experiences by writing about them. We are especially grateful to Dr. Anthony Bellissimo and Dr. Harold Merskey for their helpful advice. We are grateful to our colleagues at the Pain Clinic for their unabated support, encouragement and enthusiasm sustained over many years which contributed much in molding our ideas for the book. Our secretaries Gloria Staples and Joyce McKay made this project possible by undertaking responsibilities well beyond their call of duty. Our families showed much patience with us but at the same time provided us with encouragement, ideas, and hope, and for that we dedicate this book to our families. Finally, we wish to express our genuine appreciation of and affection for Dr. John

Basmajian, a friend and colleague, who inspires all who come to know him, and in this regard we consider ourselves highly privileged and very fortunate indeed. We would like to end on a personal note. Our names appear in alphabetical order due to its convenience.

R. ROY
E. TUNKS

Contributors

Susan Baptiste, Reg. O.T.
Director, Department of Occupational Therapy, Chedoke-McMaster Hospital, McMaster Division, Hamilton, Ontario, Canada

Darryl Bassett, M.B.
Research Fellow, Royal Adelaide Hospital, Adelaide, South Australia

Anthony Bellissimo, Ph.D.
Associate Professor, Department of Psychiatry, McMaster University, Hamilton, Ontario, Canada

Roy Cameron, Ph.D.
Associate Professor, Department of Psychology, University of Saskatchewan, Saskatoon, Saskatchewan, Canada

Joan Crook, B.S., M.A., R.N.
Associate Professor, School of Nursing, Faculty of Health Sciences, McMaster University, Hamilton, Ontario, Canada

Eugene B. Gallagher, Ph.D.
Professor, Department of Behavioral Science, University of Kentucky, Lexington, Kentucky

Edith Herman, D.P.T., M.H.Sc.
Physiotherapist, Chedoke-McMaster Hospital, McMaster Division, Hamilton, Ontario, Canada

Harold Merskey, D.M., M.R.C.P., F.R.C.P.(C), F.R.C. Psych.
Professor, Department of Psychiatry, University of Western Ontario, London Psychiatric Hospital, London, Ontario, Canada

S. Mohamed, M.D.
Director, Division of Psychiatry, Royal Inland Hospital, Kamloops, British Columbia

Issy Pilowsky, M.D.

Professor, Department of Psychiatry, University of Adelaide, Royal Adelaide Hospital, Adelaide, South Australia

Ranjan Roy, Adv. Dip. S.W.

Associate Professor, School of Social Work and Department of Psychiatry, University of Manitoba, Winnipeg, Manitoba, Canada

Eldon Tunks, M.D.

Associate Professor, Department of Psychiatry and Director, Pain Clinic, Chedoke-McMaster Hospital, Hamilton, Ontario, Canada

Anita Violon, Ph.D.

Professor, Clinique Neurochissurgicale, Rue Heger Bordet, 1 Bruxelles, Belgium

E. M. Waring, M.D.

Associate Professor, Department of Psychiatry, University of Western Ontario, London, Ontario, Canada

Sylvia Wrobel, M.A.

Department of Behavioral Science
University of Kentucky
Lexington, Kentucky

Contents

Philosophical and Conceptual Issues

Sociocultural Perspectives

Treatment Strategies

Future Directions

1

The Chronic Pain Patient and the Environment

RANJAN ROY, Adv. Dip. S.W.
ANTHONY BELLISSIMO, Ph.D.
ELDON TUNKS, M.D.

The understanding and treatment of chronic pain is a challenge faced by many health and rehabilitation professionals. The practitioner working in special clinics is confronted daily with chronic pain as a major complaint and must deal with it without a comprehensive conceptual framework that leads to an understanding of the pain in a unified way. By the time the patient arrives at the Pain Clinic, he has usually lived in that condition for a substantial length of time. The etiological factors are buried under a variety of radiographic, neurological, orthopaedic and, sometimes, psychological investigation. The patient tends to believe that he has a serious physical disability. If only the disease can be removed, he will resume his normal living! Unfortunately, some patients will not prove to have a disease to be removed or pain that can be relieved. The cost of the condition of chronic pain is incalculable in terms of social and emotional impairment and in terms of multiple medical intervention.

The effects of prolonged disability associated with chronic pain are psychological, social, economic and familial. Removal of pain is often a difficult goal for the patient with chronic pain. Not infrequently, the rationale for intervention with these patients can be sought in terms of enabling them to develop a more effective way of coping and the restoration of roles and functions, which tend to be discarded as the patient assumes his semi-invalid role. Here we see the polarity between the medical model and the rehabilitative viewpoint. The first is to eradicate the disease that causes the complaint, whereas the latter takes the complaint as the unit of concern.

1

Problem of Diverse Terminologies and Conceptual Models

On scanning the literature currently available on the subject of pain and chronic pain, it is evident that there is an enormous body of data and the developments, at least in some fields such as the neurophysiology of pain, are occurring at such a fast pace that papers written 2 years ago may be significantly out of date. Because of the breadth of the subject of pain, workers from many different medical and nonmedical disciplines are busy at work, each applying his own language and theoretical framework. It is not surprising, therefore, that some difficulty might be encountered in providing conceptual frameworks that might unify the understanding of pain. This chapter is devoted to a discussion of psychological and social factors relating to the rehabilitation of the patient with chronic pain and a discussion of conceptual models. Certainly, this narrows the field, but the problem of unifying terminology and conceptual models remains (8, 15, 16, 24).

TRADITIONAL CONCEPTUALIZATIONS

An overview of the major behavioral foundations for understanding chronic pain leads to a conclusion that there is no shortage of rationale for clinical practice. Briefly, the dominant theories of only a few decades ago were those based on the psychodynamic structure and function that had arisen from the work of Sigmund Freud and on concepts that were largely based on the medical model epitomized by the work of Kraeplin. The application of psychoanalytic theory to an understanding of pain probably reached its peak in the famous paper by Engel (7).

These psychodynamic models take an introspective approach, and the focus is upon the pain experienced, vis-a-vis, the individual's previous experience toward significant others during growth and development, the current pattern of conflicts, significant relationships, and particular personality structures. These approaches generally search for the "why," but, except for a few cases which have been worked through in laborious detail, they have not been highly productive in the alleviation of pain. The alternative to psychodynamic theories was the medical model, and without doubt the past century has been a heyday of the neuropsychiatrists. The emphasis of this approach has been primarily one of taxonomy and the maintenance of the concept of hysteria. Doubtless, many went so far as to hope that eventually, with the further development of neurological science, everything would be understandable in terms of neurophysiology and alterations of it. The natural product of such polarity in models was to perpetuate a tendency to reductionism at either pole of what appeared to be opposites: the neurological and the psychological.

PERIOD OF TRANSITION

Mid-century, a few individuals began to set a course divergent from the two mainstreams. Beecher (4) in his extensive studies of pain was certainly looking at the psychological meaning of pain, but not necessarily couched within traditional psychoanalytic understanding. He brought a pragmatic and functional emphasis which considered the meaningfulness of pain with respect to the context. Szasz (25) was, at the same time, working from his psychoanalytic training and using an object relations model. Although he was starting at a different point of observation, he was heading in the same direction in considering pain not only as a private experience but also as a communication. He considered pain to be not only a sensation but also an affect (or emotion) aroused in the context of threat. With both Beecher and Szasz then, one can see the shift toward contextual and operational definitions of pain, resting on neither the exclusive psychodynamic nor biological positions.

DEVELOPMENT OF BEHAVIORAL SCHOOLS

A new revolution in the understanding of behavior came with the development of various "behavioral schools." The antecedents of behavioristic theories were to be found in the work of Pavlov (18) and Watson (26), but the popular application of these ideas came with writers such as Wolpe (27), Lazarus (11) and Rotter (22). The central focus of behavioristic theories was to consider behavior in its own right, regardless of what events might be presumed to occur in the "black box" of the mind. The focus was to study the relationship between behavior and the events in the environment which seem to act as cues or reinforcers. These models, although no longer introspective, were nevertheless causal and were definitely contextual. Further development in these areas led to the application of learning principles to the control of events that might be considered "autonomic" (10, 17) and the biofeedback movement. Eventually, because of the particular application of these methods to disorders which had long been considered "psychosomatic" and medical, those involved in these lines of study began to see themselves as practicing "behavioral medicine" (5). The central thesis of students and practitioners of these methods is that change in behavior and personal function can be, to a great extent, altered through self-regulation. This is a process of becoming aware, responding to cues and reinforcers, and changing responses through an act of volition and awareness.

THE PAST DECADE

In the past 10 years, interactional and social theories have also become much more prominent in the behavioral sciences in general and in pain studies in particular. Thus, for example, transactional analysis as one particular model of understanding interactional communication has been employed to understand and to treat problems of chronic pain (9, 23). The interactional and social models tend to focus on the here-and-now and are not so much causal in emphasis as they are oriented toward action and response; such models are operational. Operational definitions of such things as "conversion neurosis" have also been sought from a much more sociological than psychodynamic point of view, so that we have the work of Pilowsky (19) and Pilowsky and co-workers (20, 21). This is a sociological viewpoint, originally elaborated by Mechanic (12), dealing with categories of behavior that in another terminology might have been called "hypochondriacal," "hysterical," "conversion neurosis," "dissociative" and so on. The sociological emphasis does not use introspection to search for the "why" but rather looks at the characteristics and consequences of the behavior and the role that it may play in interpersonal economy in the case of disease.

It seems that a natural outgrowth of behavioral theories based on concepts of "operant" and "classical conditioning" has been that some investigators would surely eventually ask "What exactly is going on in the black box when behavioral changes occur?" Cognitive therapy, or cognitive-behavioral therapy, has had a number of proponents including Beck (3) and Meichenbaum (13) and their students. The essential tenets have been that to understand changing behavior, one must indeed describe the behavior exactly and the context of cues and reinforcers in which it occurs. However, to have a sufficient understanding of why behavior occurs in the way it does, one must consider the thoughts that accompany it. Furthermore, certain manners and habits of thinking can be elucidated in adaptive and in maladaptive behavioral situations. From these it ought to be possible to construct learning situations in which more adaptive thinking processes can be adapted, leading to more adaptive behavior. This approach combines some aspects of introspection with the pragmatic and contextual approaches of behavioral thinking. This development can accommodate the notion that pain does not simply reflect bodily damage but is influenced by attention, anxiety, suggestion, prior conditioning, and other contextual and cognitive variables.

A recent trend which later will prove to be very important and will eventually receive a great deal of attention is that work which is being carried out by Craig (6) on the effects of modeling on pain behavior. The importance of modeling in the area of learning has been systematically explored by Bandura (1, 2) for more than a decade. Here again, the context receives major attention and the approach is operational rather than introspective, dealing with behavior as a function of apparent behavior of others in the same situation.

THEMES FOR INTEGRATION

From the above discussion, it is evident that a large number of models are becoming available for the study of pain. However, it seems that each model speaks to only part of the available data and each tends to use an esoteric language, adding to the difficulty of making accommodations between one and the other model. It is not the first time that such a point has been made with respect to pain. Beecher (4) has made similar observations. Merskey and Spear (16) suggested that a more unifying conception of pain should be adopted and proposed the definition that "Pain is an unpleasant experience felt specifically within the body and its parts and associated or usually associated with injury to the body." Sternbach (24) proposed in the concluding chapter of his book *Pain: A Psychophysiological Analysis* that pain should be considered a unitary experience modulated by a variety of factors all at the same time: factors such as the perceptual, affective, contextual, personality structure, biological, social, etc. The major efforts of these contributors have been directed toward unifying the understanding of pain, by focusing on the fact that it is a unitary whole experience and that speaking of psychological or biological events, for example, is to make abstractions. Only the pain itself, in its totality, is not an abstraction.

Despite efforts of such persons as Sternbach and Merskey to encourage unifying conceptualizations of pain, a number of factors mitigate against the process of bringing unity and compatibility between models and observations. One factor is the wealth of biological and behavioral data which is simply becoming overwhelming, so that the acquisition of knowledge is happening at a rate, it seems, faster than it can be assimilated and put into perspective. A second factor relates to an intuitive notion, which still remains, that pain is within a physical body and usually arises in the presence of physical damage. Thus, there is a ready temptation to look for a physical cause or, abandoning that, retreat to a completely psychological cause (despite the fact that to call pain a "physical" or "psychological" event is, in both cases, to deal with only part of the data). The third factor is the nature of medical practice itself, with its various disciplines divided among psychological and nonpsychological lines. There is no medical discipline that is formally devoted to the integrative understanding of human distress. Many practitioners of "holistic" medicine are divorced from any scientific base. Psychiatric disciplines may lay claim to having eclectic practitioners but still operate in a medical milieu which streams patients and their handling into psychological and nonpsychological compartments. Therefore, because of these three factors—the wealth of accumulating data, intuitive notions of pain, and the professional milieu—the clinician still may be forced to adopt an either/or attitude toward the clinical problems of chronic pain. The way this occurs in practice, for example, is that an individual may be diagnosed as suffering from pain due to a certain "medical" cause but "with a psychological overlay." Such thinking acknowledges the behavioral aspects of the problem almost as an afterthought. The equivalent sort of reasoning exists when the diagnosis of "psychogenic pain" is made, but with the additional concession that certain psychophysiological events naturally accompany the primary psychogenic process. In this latter case, the physical aspects of the problem are added almost as an afterthought. The clinician may also retreat to reductionistic approaches such as the overoptimistic "neurologizing," for example, in taking the gate theory of pain (14) beyond what it was designed to do in attempting to medically legitimize complicated pain problems.

To summarize the argument at this point, it can be seen that there is a variety of psychological and social models available for description of chronic pain, and each model takes into account only part of the data available. Each tends to use a language which makes resolution of differences between models and integration of these viewpoints difficult. There has been the development of an awareness of this problem over recent years. This appears to be reflected in the occurrence of some of the new models of behavior such as the cognitive-behavioral therapy model which tries to account not only for behavior in its context but also for events within the individual, combining introspection with a pragmatic look at the whole. There has been a definite trend away from compartmentalizing and away from the old body-mind dichotomy. The focus, instead, is on giving priority of consideration to the clinical problem itself and on recognizing that any models applied deal with parts of the whole. Attempts to develop a taxonomy of pain are part of this effort (15). In addition, models that are being developed are recognizing that the major benefit is not going to result from theories which question "why?" in a deterministic way, such as is the case with psychoanalytic theory. It is expected that advances are going to be made by theories which recognize the occurrence of the event in its context and make sense of it there, looking at the utility of certain behaviors and styles of adaptation and at the response that such behaviors bring. There-fore, the thrust is toward an ecological, adaptive and operational emphasis and away from a post-hoc hypothesizing regarding antecedents of a given event or behavior. It is the above recent developments and the argument outlined that serve as the major thrust of this book.

Organization of the Book

The chapters that follow elaborate some of the themes presented in this introductory chapter. The concluding chapter will re-address the theme of the development of a new conceptual language of chronic pain and the ecological adaptive thesis. Between the introductory and the concluding chapters, three general sections can be identified: 1) philosophical issues and definitions (Chapters 2 and 3), 2) sociological perspective (Chapters 4, 5 and 6) and 3) intervention.

In Chapters 2 and 3, some of the philosophical issues and definitions as they relate to the chronic pain problem are discussed. Specifically, Chapter 2 considers the body-mind dilemma and the problems created by our medical language. It discusses the nature of pain and looks at pain associated with major physical lesions and pain associated with minor or no physical lesions. Chapter 3 deals with the process of becoming a chronic pain patient. It highlights the problem of pain as a nonspecific disorder, challenges the notion of "no disease, no pain," and suggests a "medical way" of resolving the problem.

The sociological perspective is discussed in Chapters 4, 5 and 6. They deal with particular theoretical issues which must be considered in any under-standing of the psychological and sociological implications of chronic pain. Chapter 4 discusses the chronic sick role as a "tolerated deviance" or "socially accepted dependency." Similar to the view expressed in Chapter 3, the problem of legitimizing chronic pain is identified. However, here the discussion is directed toward the Pain Clinic as a new social structure whose function is the "medicalization" of chronic pain, with certain corollaries. Chapter 5 looks at the neglected area of the patient and the role of work. It takes an ecological view and focuses on how the occupational role is central to the role of the adult male (note the different emphasis for women in Chapter 6) and how work has been used as a cardinal criterion for successful treatment outcome. In discussing the female patient with chronic pain, Chapter 6 builds on the argument that our philosophical assumptions, in part, determine what we do. It presents an historical discussion of societal attitudes toward women in pain, focusing on the continued presence of the notion of women as being victims of biological constraints. This bias regard-ing women is present in societal structures set up to assist disabled people. It would be easy to describe the injured worker who has become a chronic pain patient as a malingerer or a "compensation-seeker" and the woman's issue as feminism. The importance of the three chapters in this section lies in the examination of familiar attitudes and the social environment as participants in the illness event.

Intervention is the main concern of Chapters 7 through 13. They deal with behavioral and cognitive psychotherapy, individual psychotherapy, conjoint and family therapy, and consultation psychiatry, respectively. Chapter 7 presents a critical review of the research and clinical literature in the areas of behavior therapy, cognitive therapy and biofeedback. It also discusses the process of integrating these approaches in their application to chronic pain. Chapter 8, by Drs. Pilowsky and Basset, builds on the psycho-dynamic understanding of the person as well as on the wealth of wisdom that comes from much experience in treating chronic pain patients and studying their problems. It is valuable to note that the perspectives con-tained in Chapter 8 are not simply self-evident conclusions drawn from conventional psychiatric concepts, but rather they illustrate the knowledge and skill that must be acquired first-hand in managing chronic pain. Chapter 9 argues for conceptualizing individual psychotherapy in a broader context than the traditional (psychodynamic) methods and positions. Two chapters, 10 and 11, deal with particular application of the psychology of family systems to the understanding and treatment of pain problems. Chapter 11 further offers several examples of such analysis and therapy. Particular attention is given to the idea of "cognitive family therapy" as one particular approach that seems to be effective in helping families of patients who suffer chronic pain. Within an overview of group psychotherapy, Chapter 12 presents a particular application of group therapy in chronic pain. The program described evolved specifically from work with pain patients and has especial relevance to this work. With reference to the results of a group experience, the effective ingredients are discussed. The work of the psychiatrist who is a consultant to the rehabilitation unit or pain clinic is the subject of the 13th chapter. Probably this has received less than adequate attention in recent literature, notwithstanding valuable contributions from the point of view of psychology and "behavioral medicine." The final chapter is directed toward synthesis and summarizes the two essential theses of this book. The first is that our language needs to be revised and unified and our conceptual models need to be considered in light of each other in such a way that dichotomizing will no longer contaminate clear thinking about chronic pain. The second is that advances in our understanding will not easily occur with only the introspective and post-hoc models which ask "Why did this behavior occur?" It will occur with models that address the questions, "What is the context of this problem?", "How is the problem defined operationally in terms of its context?", "How can adaptation be defined?" and "What commonalities can be discovered when pain persists or changes?" We will never eliminate from society the causes for chronic pain but must seek answers to the question "What are the psychosocial factors essential to successful rehabilitation?"

REFERENCES

1. BANDURA, A. *Social Learning Theory.* Prentice-Hall, Englewood Cliffs, N.J., 1977.
2. BANDURA, A., AND WALTERS, R. H. *Social Learning and Personality Development.* Holt, Rinehart and Winston, New York, 1963.
3. BECK, A. T. *Cognitive Therapy and the Emotional Disorders.* International University Press, New York, 1976.
4. BEECHER, H. K. Relationship of significance of wound to pain experienced. *J. A. M. A., 161:* 1609–1613, 1956.
5. BIRK, L. *Biofeedback: Behavioral Medicine.* Grune and Stratton, New York, 1973.
6. CRAIG, K. D. Social modeling influences on pain. In *The Psychology of Pain,* edited by R. A. Sternbach, Raven Press, New York, pp. 73–109, 1978.
7. ENGEL, G. L. Psychogenic pain and the pain prone patient. *Am. J. Med., 26:* 849–918, 1959.
8. FORDYCE, W. E. *Behavioral Methods for Chronic Pain and Illness.* C. V. Mosby, St. Louis, 1976.
9. GREENHOOT, J. H., AND STERNBACH, R. A. Conjoint treatment of chronic pain. In *Advances in Neurology, Vol 4: Pain,* edited by J. J. Bonica. Raven Press, New York, pp. 595–603, 1974.
10. KATKIN, E. S., AND MURRAY, E. N. Instrumental conditioning of autonomically mediated behavior: Theoretical and methodological issues. *Psychol. Bull, 70:* 52–68, 1978.
11. LAZARUS, A. A. New methods in psychotherapy: A case study. *South African Med. J., 33:* 660–663, 1958.
12. MECHANIC, D. *Medical Sociology: A Selective View.* Free Press, New York, 1968.
13. MEICHENBAUM, D. H. *Cognitive-Behavior Modification: An Integrative Approach.* Plenum Press, New York, 1977.
14. MELZACK, R. *The Puzzle of Pain.* Basic Books, New York, 1973.
15. MERSKEY, H., et al. Pain terms: A list with definitions and notes on usage. Recommended by the IASP subcommittee on Taxonomy. *Pain, 6:* 249–252; 1979.

16. MERSKEY, H., AND SPEAR, F. G. *Pain: Psychological and Psychiatric Aspects.* Balliere, Tindall, and Cassell, London, 1967.
17. MILLER, N. E. Learning of visceral and glandular responses. *Science, 163:* 434–455, 1969.
18. PAVLOV, I. P. *Lectures on Conditioned Reflexes.* International Publishers, New York, 1928.
19. PILOWSKY, I. Abnormal illness behavior. *Br. J. Med. Psychol., 42:* 347–351, 1969.
20. PILOWSKY, I., CHAPMAN, C. R., AND BONICA, J. J. Pain, depression, and illness behavior in a pain clinic population. *Pain, 4:* 183–189, 1977.
21. PILOWSKY, I., AND SPENCE, N. Pain and illness behavior: A comparative study. *J. Psychosom. Res., 30:* 131–134, 1976.
22. ROTTER, J. B. *Social Learning and Clinical Psychology.* Prentice-Hall, Englewood Cliffs, N.J., 1954.
23. STERNBACH, R. A. Varieties of pain games. In J. J. BONICA (Ed.), *Advances in Neurology, Vol. 4: Pain.* Raven Press, New York, 1974, pp. 423–432.
24. STERNBACH, R. A. *Pain: A Psychophysiological Analysis.* Academic Press, New York, 1968.
25. SZASZ, T. S. The nature of pain. *Arch. Neurol. Psychiatry, 74:* 174–181, 1955.
26. WATSON, J. B. Psychology as the behaviorist views it. *Psychol. Rev., 20:* 158–177, 1913.
27. WOLPE, J. *Psychotherapy by Reciprocal Inhibition.* Stanford University Press, Stanford, CA, 1958.

2

Body-Mind Dilemma in Chronic Pain

H. MERSKEY, D.M., M.R.C.P., F.R.C.P.(C), F.R.C.Psych.

This chapter deals with two issues. The first is the nature of pain or what we mean by pain and how we define it. The second is the difference between people who have pain which is related to major physical lesions and those who have pain with little or no physical disturbance.

The particular position which I adopt is based on philosophical arguments advanced by T.S. Szasz (36), some of whose other views I often think perverse. However, in regard to this topic Szasz has stated a position which allows us to establish what can be called pain. This in turn permits us to escape the needless snares of the body-mind dilemma.

According to some philosophers, e.g., Bertrand Russell (33), there are two types of data: public data which we can all in principle observe and private data which are limited to the individual. Public data comprise items like "There is a black cat crossing the road." Assuming reasonable vision, normal visibility, and adequate proximity to the object, all observers can agree (or disagree) with the statement. The events in question are outside all the observers and their occurrence is confirmed or not confirmed empirically by valid tests.

Private data are in a different class because they depend on a report from subjective experience to which the only person who has access is the individual who issues the report. "I feel happy" may be said by a man who looks lugubrious and there is no way to deny his statement. We may suspect he is not giving us a true report of his feelings, and if he goes on to commit suicide we may wonder if he was being honest with us. However, no one else can directly confirm or deny his claim. "I have a pain" is a statement of the same type. So long as he is telling the truth, no one else can dispute it. We may be inclined to believe him readily if his leg is broken and he shows external manifestations of pain such as dilated pupils, shock and pallor. On the other hand, we may wonder about his bona fides or at least his accuracy if he lays claim to severe pain whilst in a smiling and apparently relaxed state. But there is no way by which we can, ultimately, challenge his report of his private experience. The point is that pain is a subjective event which we do (or do not) experience. Subjective events are not observable by anyone except the person who experiences them. The observation of a black cat, or a ginger one for that matter, is also a subjective event. However, since its occurrence is placed outside the observer, others may check whether a comparable event is generated in them. This is not so with pain, which is an experience of something internal no matter how it is produced. Such internal events are always described in the language of experience— that is to say, in the language of psychology. External events, public data, are described ultimately in the language of physics, which presupposes the possibility of an external observer checking what takes place. Perhaps it is hard for us to recognize that pain is always an internal event because we naturally conceive of it as so often being produced by external forces.

There are of course numerous physical events which can be associated with reports of the subjective experience of pain. Some of these such as broken limbs and changes in appearance have already been mentioned. A swollen and inflamed fingertip, a gouty toe, a gastric ulcer and an accumulation of gallstones in the gall bladder, with perhaps one in the common bile duct, all have a frequent but not invariable relationship to reports of pain. Yet such events only serve to make a report of pain more acceptable to us. They do not prove its occurrence. Similarly, many fascinating changes may be observed in the nervous system after stimuli which we normally consider may cause pain. Nerve cells which react only to damaging, noxious stimuli can be demonstrated in animal studies (18). Operations upon portions of the nervous system may abolish the pain which would otherwise be anticipated from noxious stimuli in a given area. Damage to parts of the brain or to peripheral nerves may induce intractable pain. All this, as well as common experience, seems to suggest that pain is a consequence of physical changes in the body, and it is not to be denied.

It follows that there is a temptation to describe pain as the physical changes which result from noxious stimulation or from malfunction of those parts of the nervous system which normally respond to such events. As a corollary, patients who do not have lesions but do have pain are liable to be considered as not "genuine." It is at this point that the distinction between private and public data becomes useful or important to us. The changes in the nervous system may be observed in principle, if not often in practice, by more than one observer and sometimes may be recorded on a cathode ray tube. The changes in the individual's experience remain his alone to report. If the changes in the nervous system persist during general anesthesia, they may be observed by a whole team of experimenters or operators, but if the individual is adequately asleep and oblivious to those changes (even though his blood pressure rises and he groans and his muscles twitch) and if afterwards he reports no memory of pain, we can never say that he had any. Certainly he had changes in the nervous system characteristic of those which we would anticipate in an individual in pain, but pain was absent. This extreme position can occasionally be paralled in patients who are awake and who undergo impressive trauma with no pain or with much less pain than we would anticipate (2, 4, 28, 34).

In correspondence with the above, if individuals report pain without lesions and without observable nervous system changes, they must normally be supposed to have pain. The risk of life or health from such pain is likely to be less than in people who have lesions. Associated generalized physiological change may well be less or different (20) but the individuals still subjectively have pain, and their report of their private experience remains the ground for that conclusion.

Pain Without Lesions

A number of people—how many and in what proportion is unknown—appear to have pain in the absence of a physical cause. Others have pain which is made worse by emotional factors. Evidence on this score is to be found in the volumes already cited (28, 34, 40) and elsewhere in this volume. For many authors, this has presented a problem. If there is no lesion, how can there be pain? I am not suggesting that we have satisfactory answers to that question. The most extreme examples are provided by patients who appear to develop pain as a result of thought processes, e.g., an interne reported by Beck (3) who experienced pain in his own sternum when about to take a sternal marrow from a patient. The couvade syndrome—pains in men during their wives' labors or pregnancies—is another example. Patients with no discernible physical basis for their pain are encountered in clinical practice with a frequency which depends somewhat upon the sample of patients and the selection patterns but occur sufficiently often to be known to almost all clinicians. I have reviewed elsewhere (25, 26) the idea that pain may arise purely from thought processes. Some suggestions have been made that pain may arise as a result of an hallucination (although rarely) or as a consequence of a muscle tension mechanism. Hallucinations are sensory experiences, in such illnesses as schizophrenia, in which there is no external stimulus to cause the experience. In the case of muscle tension we are really postulating a psychosomatic effect with a physical basis for the pain, but this may be a less-sound explanation than is often believed. The idea of thought processes causing pain has been linked in some instances to hysterical mechanisms (25). The latter involve the occurrence of a symptom as a result of unconscious thought processes. Hallucination or hysterical mechanisms require no physical lesion. In the case of muscle tension there may be a physiological mechanism involved. In all cases the patients describe their experience in two fundamental ways: first, they say that it is unpleasant—it hurts—and they indicate that they conceive of it as an experience related to bodily trauma or change in the tissues. The words they use to describe pain are such as "stinging," "aching," "burning," "throbbing," "pressing," "like a knife," and so forth. There are some differences between patients with lesions and those without lesions (1, 32). Those without lesions use slightly more evaluative or affect-laden words, but the descriptions of pain by psychiatric patients overall are notable for their similarity to those of the physically ill (1, 11, 15).

Thus we have to accept that the two main aspects of pain as an experience are 1) that it is unpleasant (in a characteristic way) and 2) that we associate it with tissue damage. These characteristics are recognized in the definition of pain adopted by the International Association for the Study of Pain (1979) which is "an unpleasant sensory and emotional experience which is associated with tissue damage or described in terms of tissue damage." This definition represents a conscious decision of its advocates that we can only call pain something which is part of the subjective experience of an individual. Actual changes in tissue and in the nervous system are not pain.

We first learn to identify pain as a distinct experience when we suffer trauma or some illness and are told that the particular experience (a bruised knee as a child, a sore throat after tonsillectomy) is called pain. Thereafter, those experiences which we associate with trauma or physiological dysfunction are recognized as painful and are described in appropriate words (29). Nothing else is pain.

The Disappearance of the Dilemma

At this point the mind-body dilemma vanishes as if in a conjuring trick. This is because we cease to confuse the subjective, private experience with the external verifiable events. We have made a distinction between the language of physiology or physics and that of psychology. The events of the mind come into the latter domain. What we are doing is employing two languages for different aspects of the same events. We are using two different sorts of descriptions, neither parallel nor dichotomous nor interacting but alternative for the same occurrences. Philosophically this position is known as monism. It preserves the separate languages which are useful and does not confuse private phenomena described in the one language with publicly observable phenomena in the other. It is a sort of bilingualism or coding, in which the words of one language or code are not usable in the other language but in which they will correspond to each other and describe the same events. In regard to pain the correspondence is not absolute; if it were, we would know enough to specify all the physiological changes which occur when an individual says he has pain or does not have pain, whether these are or are not lesions which would normally be expected to produce pain. In principle, however, the correspondence is complete because we are describing the same events in different terms. In practice, psychological terms are often better descriptions than are physiological terms or else are more usable. The sensations from a gouty toe or limb are poorly described for most people, and inaccurately for all, as a lesion of such and such a size with so and so many impulses per second being generated from it in X number of nerve terminals—they are described much better as a jabbing needle-like pain.

If pain is treated always as an experience, one of the consequences is that we do not require to establish its cause in order to recognize or describe its occurrence. All subjective events which share the common qualities of being unpleasant and capable of description in terms of trauma, noxious stimulation, damage or distortion of tissues will be pain. It follows that we cannot assume that there are two *types* of pain which are somehow different: "psychogenic" and "organic" pain, the first perhaps a little less genuine than the second. There is only pain. The pain may have different recognizable causes (lesions, physiological dysfunction, emotional problems, behavioral reinforcement or some mixture of all of these) but the important causes do not define the existence of pain; they do, however, help to account for it when it happens.

It also follows from what has been said that it is not advisable to talk of pain as "psychogenic" or "organic." The use of these terms may blur a complex situation in which several causes are operating. More important, the use of the terms "psychogenic" and "organic" tends to lead to discrimination between two types of patient, the one being regarded as less "genuine" than the other. Thirdly, and not without weight, it has been noted by Lewis (21) that the word "psychogenic" itself has changed in meaning several times in English and in German. Initially in English it was used in the context of biological disputes and appears to have had evolutionary connotations. Later in German it meant a psychological condition with various causes, including constitutional predisposition and suggestibility. The meaning changed by several shades with different German authorities and no unanimity was achieved for it. Lewis quotes one Scandinavian author of recent date as saying that "psychogenic can refer equally well to something caused or produced by the psyche as to some alteration in the psyche due to situational or environmental—particularly interpersonal— factor." Lewis concludes that the term is better dropped, and I agree with this. We do have to recognize, however, when describing pain that it is important to indicate what we think its main causes are, and so one has to distinguish at least at times between pain which depends mainly or wholly on psychological factors and pain which depends mainly or wholly on organic factors. This is more cumbersome than the old terms, but it is also more careful.

Psychological Causes and Effects of Pain

It has been indicated so far that pain may result from psychological causes, and three mechanisms were suggested whereby this may occur. The recognition that a pain located in the body may arise for psychological reasons is very old. What gives it force right up to the present time is the daily experience of clinicians who encounter patients with persistent pain for which no organic explanation is satisfactory and with evidence of emotional factors which appear to cause the pain. The evidence is not always forthcoming, but when it is and when the pain is relieved by psychiatric treatment it becomes reasonable to accept that the prime factor producing the somatic experience is an emotional one. A woman who was unhappy in her marriage experienced sustained headache until she left her husband. It then cleared up completely until she met him for a discussion and it recovered again at the end of their meeting. Such anecdotal evidence is supported by many reports which indicate that the emotional disturbance which is found in many patients with chronic pain is disproportionate to their physical lesions. For example, Walters (40) reported 430 patients with chronic pain many of whom had lesions, where the pain was increased as a result of emotional factors. Merskey (23, 24) described 100 psychiatric patients with chronic pain seen in a period of approximately 3 years in routine psychiatric practice, amongst whom only 2 had a significant organic cause for pain and 4 had a minor possible cause; if the psychiatric illness was effectively treatable, improvement in the pain occurred. Bradley (7) showed that pain appearing with depression in 19 patients remitted with recovery. Unfortunately, there is a hard core of patients with chronic pain and insufficient evidence of physical illness who show only limited responses to psychiatric treatment. They tend to have hypochondriacal or hysterical characteristics and some depression. On psychological testing the pattern of the "conversion V triad" is found using the Minnesota Multiphasic Personality Inventory (MMPI), i.e., elevations by one or two standard deviations on the hypochondriasis (Hs) and hysteria (Hy) scales and a slightly lesser elevation of the depression (D) scale. Pilling et al. (31) noted it in patients with pain as a presenting symptom. Sternbach (35) summarizes the evidence for this pattern, and Hanvik (16) and many others (6, 9, 19, 41, 42) have also found it with low back pain.

The most classical example of pain due to emotional causes is Effort Syndrome, in which pain, difficulty in breathing, and fatigue are all found. It was first described in 1871 by DaCosta (10) in a man who also had an aphonia which DaCosta called catarrhal but which lasted 8 months, cleared up spontaneously and was presumably hysterical. Effort Syndrome has been a well-recognized response of soldiers to the stress of military service or battle, and chest pain without any organic basis is nearly always found as part of it, whilst a clear psychological cause is evident. Still other examples of pain arising without organic disease and with evident psychological cause include innumerable examples of tension headache and vascular headache (14). At least the first of these two types of headache is primarily emotional in origin and the second one is often held to be so.

For our purposes in this chapter it is sufficient to recognize the following: patients without organic lesions may have pain because of anxiety and depression. It may appear in association with personality disorder, especially one with hysterical, histrionic or dependent characteristics, and there are several possible psychological mechanisms to which it may be attributed. However, we also need to consider the way in which pain arising from gross lesions may affect the emotional status of the individual.

The Effect of Pain

The increasing attention which has been paid to emotional factors causing pain has led in the past few years to some neglect of the possibility that physical illness, and especially sustained noxious input, might be emotionally harmful to individuals. Yet, it should have been obvious that continued severe pain might be damaging to the personality. We do not often see this as clearly in our ordinary practice as was the case in the past when methods of relieving pain were not so readily available or so efficient. However, it was known to Weir Mitchell, amongst others, as the following quotation indicated. Describing a man who had sustained a causalgic lesion he wrote, "From being a man of gay and kindly temper, known in his company as a good natured jester, he became morose and melancholy and complained that reading gave him vertigo, and that his memory of recent events was bad." The neurosurgeon Livingston (22) was another author who recognized the contribution of physical lesions in changing the emotional pattern of the individual. Other evidence on this topic has come from several sources. Woodforde and Merskey (43) found that patients with pain of physical origin were actually more anxious, more depressed and more subject to signs of neuroticism than were a comparison group of patients whose pain had no physical cause but who were known to have psychiatric illness. The patients with lesions had high L scores on the Eysenck Personality Inventory. This may be interpreted as indicating that they believe themselves once to have been people who were well adjusted and emotionally stable and who functioned well but felt that now they were different. This is certainly the impression we have had in talking with some of them. Other authors (5, 30) have found a rise in the L scale among the physically ill. It appears that individuals who are aware of damage to their personalities and know that they have become subject to increasing anxiety and depression attribute the changes to the chronic pain from which they are suffering. It also appears that the L scale is perhaps not, as so-called, a "lie scale" but one which reflects the effect of chronic illness.

The effects of chronic illness were also demonstrated by Crown and Crown (8), who compared patients with early and late rheumatoid arthritis. Those with newly developed rheumatoid arthritis were not particularly neurotic, but those whose illnesses had been present for some time showed more evidence of emotional change. We can reasonably conclude that chronic noxious stimulation experienced with pain is associated with alterations of personality. Some of these alterations of personality may be in the direction of irritability. Biological evidence of irritability and aggression in response to noxious stimulation has been shown by Ulrich et al. (38) and Ulrich (37), who demonstrated that aggression is a frequent response to trauma. When rats were given electric shocks through the floors of their cages, they would turn and bite their neighbors. Such aggression can be thought of as part of a "fight or flight mechanism." Normally, we assume that the main biological value of pain is in securing rest which leads to healing (17) or leads us to take other measures to protect and cure lesions. However, the alternative biological value should not be neglected, and that is to prepare or to alert the individual to the need for self-defense. When pain affects the viscera, it is probably too late for fighting to become an effective defense against a cause of pain. Characteristically, visceral pain is heavy and sickening and leads to immediate withdrawal from activity. On the other hand, cutaneous pain which will arise with relatively minor damage to the body and to its surfaces is more behaviorally stimulating, may be sexually arousing (12, 13), and may prepare the individual more for fighting. Thus some of the effects of pain depend upon the situation and source of pain, but they can often be seen to be biologically potent as well as psychologically important.

Similarities and Differences Between Types of Pain

In what has been said so far, no special distinction has been made between acute and chronic pain. It cannot be overemphasized that the pain requires accurate diagnosis, whether it is acute or chronic. Nevertheless, with chronic pain, despite the best efforts at diagnosis and all reasonable investigation, the position is sometimes reached that it is uncertain whether the pain is primarily physical or primarily psychological in origin or is due to an approximately equal mixture of both causes. The extreme cases, in which the causes of pain are clearly different, seem to justify this "physical versus psychological" approach to etiology. Nevertheless, some authors have approached the problem by seeing pain as having similar common factors of etiology, including psychological causes, whether or not pain was primarily due to a physical illness. For example, Violon (39) has argued that pain of cluster headache and other facial pains which may have physical causes were nevertheless much promoted in her patients by their childhood experiences.

The evidence for this is not really strong at present and more comparative data are needed. In the cases of hysterical pain compared with, for example, central pain, the contrasts between the two approaches are the most evident. However, the more one encounters the mixture of psychological and physical causes which is typical of clinical practice, the more difficult it is to sort out how much one factor is causing the pain and how much another. It is at this point that the conceptual approach offered in this chapter is perhaps maximally useful. For the mixed group of patients, in whom the pain seems the same phenomenologically even while its causes are varied, a uniform approach to their condition is the most effective in helping the patient and is the most sensible from the point of view of the physician. This approach requires an acceptance of the reality of the pain and at the same time a decision to treat from whatever direction is appropriate. Some treatment differences of course immediately follow from the distinction as to causes. Where the physical cause is predominant, or is felt to be so, phenothiazines, antidepressants, minor analgesics and occasionally (depending on the situation) narcotic analgesics may be required. In all cases, support, exploratory psychotherapy, cognitive therapy, possible behavioral management, acupuncture and a variety of psychological and semipsychological/physiological techniques may be required. It is as hard to separate treatments as to separate the theoretical causes in responding to patients with pain.

REFERENCES

1. AGNEW, D. C., AND MERSKEY, H. Words of chronic pain. *Pain, 2:* 73–81, 1976.
2. BARBER, T. X. Toward a theory of pain: Relief of chronic pain by pre-frontal leucotomy, opiates, placebos and hypnosis. *Psychol. Bull., 56:* 430–460, 1959.
3. BECK, A. T. *Cognitive Therapy and the Emotional Disorders.* International Universities Press, New York, 1967.
4. BEECHER, H. K. Relationship of significance of wound to the pain experienced. *J.A.M.A., 161:* 1609–1613, 1956.
5. BOND, M. R. The relation of pain to the Eysenck Personality Inventory, Cornell Medical Index and Whiteley Index of Hyopchondriasis. *Br. J. Psychiatry., 119:* 671–678, 1971.
6. BLUMETTI, A. E., AND MODESTI, L. M. Psychological predictors of success or failure of surgical intervention for intractable back pain. In *Advances in Pain Research and Therapy, Vol. 1,* edited by J.J. Bonica and D. Albe-Fessard. Raven Press, New York, pp. 323–325, 1976.
7. BRADLEY, J. J. Severe localized pain associated with the depressive syndrome. *Br. J. Psychiatry, 109:* 741–745, 1963.
8. CROWN, S., AND CROWN, J. M. Personality in early rheumatic disease. *J. Psychosom. Res., 17:* 189–196, 1973.
9. CUMMINGS, C., EVANSKI, P. M., DeBENDETTI, M. J., AND WAUGH, T. R. Use of the MMPI in a low back pain treatment program. *Pain Abstracts, Vol. 1., 2nd World Congress of International Association Study of Pain,* p. 247, 1978.
10. DACOSTA, J. M. On irritable heart: A clinical study of a form of functional cardiac disorder and its consequences. *Am. J. Med. Sci., 61:* 17–52, 1871.
11. DEVINE, R., AND MERSKEY, H. The description of pain in psychiatric and general medical patients. *J. Psychosom. Res., 9:* 311–316, 1965.
12. ELLIS, H. H. *Studies in the Psychology of Sex.* Random House, New York, 1936.
13. FORD, C. S., AND BEACH, F. A. *Patterns of Sexual Behaviour.* Eyre and Spottiswoode, London, 1952.
14. FRIEDMAN, A. P., FINLEY, K. H., GRAHAM, J. R., KUNKLE, C. E., OSTFELD, M. O., AND WOLFF, H. G. Classification of headache: Special report of the Ad Hoc Committee. *Arch. Neurol., 6:* 173–176, 1962.
15. GITTLESON, N. L. Psychiatric headache: A clinical study. J. Ment. Sci., *107:* 403–416, 1961.
16. HANVIK, J. L. MMPI profiles in patients with low-back pain. Article 55 from *Basic Reading on the MMPI in Psychology and Medicine,* edited by G. S. Welsh and W. G. Dahlstrom, pp. 499–504, Oxford University Press, London, 1956.

17. HILTON (1863). *Rest and Pain.* edited by W. Jacobson, George Bell & Sons. London, 3rd ed., 1880.
18. IGGO, A. The case for "pain" receptors. In *Pain,* edited by R. Janzen et al., pp. 60–77, Churchill-Livingstone, London, 1972.
19. JAMISON, K., FERRER-BRECHNER, M. T., BRECHNER, V. L., AND McCREARY, C. P. Correlation of personality profile with pain syndrome. In *Advances in Pain Research and Therapy,* Vol. 1., edited by J. J. Bonica and D. Albe-Fessard. Raven Press, New York, pp. 317–321, 1976.
20. LASCELLES, P. T., EVANS, P. R., MERSKEY, H., AND SABUR, M. A. Plasma cortisol in psychiatric and neurological patients with pain. *Brain,* 97(pt III): 533–538, 1974.
21. LEWIS, A. "Psychogenic": A word and its mutations. *Psychol. Med.,* 2: 209–215, 1972.
22. LIVINGSTON, W. K. *Pain Mechanisms: A Physiologic Interpretations of Causalgia and Its Related States.* Plenum Press, New York, 1976.
23. MERSKEY, H. The characteristics of persistent pain in psychological illness. *J. Psychosom. Res.,* 9: 291–298, 1965.
24. MERSKEY, H. Psychiatric patients with persistent pain. *J. Psychosom Res., 9:* 299–309, 1965.
24. MERSKEY, H. *The Analysis of Hysteria.* Bailliere, Tindall, London, 1974.
26. MERSKEY, H. The role of the psychiatrist in the investigation and treatment of pain. *Res. Publ. Assoc. Res. Nerv. Ment. Dis.,* 58: 249–260, 1980.
27. MERSKEY, H., et al., Pain terms: A list with definitions and notes on usage. Recommended by an International Association for the Study of Pain Subcommittee on Taxonomy. *Pain,* 6: 249–252, 1979.
28. MERSKEY, H., AND SPEAR, F. G. *Pain: Psychological and Psychiatric Aspects.* Bailliere, Tindall and Cassell, London, 1967.
29. MERSKEY, H., AND SPEAR, F. G. The concept of pain, Proceedings of 10th Annual Conference of the Society for Psychosomatic Research. *J. Psychosom. Res., 11:* 59–67, 1967.
30. MORGENSTERN, F. S. *Chronic Pain.* D.M. Thesis, Oxford, 1967.
31. PILLING, L. F., BRANNICK, T. L., AND SWENSON, W. M. Psychological characteristics of patients having pain as a presenting symptom. *Can. Med. Assoc. J.,* 97: 387–394, 1967.
32. READING, A. E., AND NEWTON, J. R. A comparison of primary dysmenorrhea and intrauterine device related pain. *Pain, 3:* 265–276, 1977.
33. RUSSELL, B. *Human Knowledge: Its Scope and Limits.* Simon and Schuster, London, 1948.
34. STERNBACH, R. A. *Pain: A Psychophysiological Analysis.* Academic Press, New York, 1968.
35. STERNBACH, R. A. *Pain Patients: Traits and Treatment.* Academic Press, New York, 1974.
36. SZASZ, T. S. *Pain and Pleasure.* Tavistock Publications, London, 1957.
37. ULRICH, R. E. Pain as a cause of aggression. *Amer. Zool.,* 6: 643, 1966.
38. ULRICH, R. E., HUTCHINSON, P. R., AND AZRIN, N. H. Pain-elicited aggression. *Psychol. Rev., 15:* 111–126, 1965.
39. VIOLON, A. *Le Syndrome Douloureux Chronique: Étude Psychologique.* Doctoral Dissertation. Free University of Brussels, 1978.
40. WALTERS, A. Psychogenic regional pain alias hysterical pain. *Brain, 84:* 1–18, 1961.
41. WARING, E. M., WEISZ, G. M., AND BAILEY, S. I. Predictive factors in the treatment of low back pain by surgical intervention. In *Advances in Pain Research and Therapy,* Vol. 1, edited by J.J. Bonica and D. Albe-Fessard. Raven Press, New York, pp. 939–942, 1976.
42. WILTSE, L. L., AND ROCCHIO, P. D. Preoperative psychological tests as predictors of success of chemonucleolysis in the treatment of low-back pain syndrome. *J. Bone Joint Surg., 57:* 478–483, 1975.
43. WOODFORDE, J. M., AND MERSKEY, H. Personality traits of psychiatric patients with chronic pain. *J. Psychosom. Res., 16:* 167–172, 1972.

3

The Process Involved in Becoming a Chronic Pain Patient

An Historical Analysis of the Problem

For almost 20 centuries, pain in occidental tradition has been considered a punishment for sin or guilt and also a means of expiation, thus of saving one's soul.

Human life in our countries has indeed been put under the seal of pain and suffering according to the doctrine of "original sin." Pain can thus be considered a malediction or a way of spiritually joining the Lord. Ecstasy has even been described in people who were burned at the stake for their religious beliefs, probably because of the prospect of salvation of their soul (14).

This ambivalent view—malediction and salvation at the same time— remains vivid now in popular tradition. For instance, French-speaking people say about an individual who has suffered much: "Il a gagné son paradis" (he won his paradise).

Thus, like depression, chronic pain is associated with the concepts of guilt and expiation, and pain can refer to a religious or neurotic experience. Nevertheless, talking about pain may be confusing; the subject we shall deal with here in fact is not pain, but pain patients.

The term "pain patients" refers to those who present with a complaint of pain, seeking relief from it (19), i.e., patients whose complaint is chronic, persisting constantly or intermittently for several months or years.

An impressive amount of literature has been devoted to pain, especially during the past decade. Very little, however, has been written about how one becomes a pain patient.

Usually, pain is only a symptom of a disease. However, when chronic, pain may be a disease in itself (2): the patient is "pain-sick."

20

CLASSICAL PSYCHODYNAMIC VIEW OF PAIN PATIENTS

Psychoanalysts on the one hand consider chronic pain as a conversion symptom resulting from unconscious psychic conflicts. According to them, bodily pain is a symbolic translation of an unpleasant affect, an hysterical conversion.

Reviewing Freud's work in regard to pain patients, Merskey and Spear (16) have stressed the usual presence of conflict, guilt and resentment in most of the cases wherein pain was a prominent symptom. Subsequent psychoanalytic contributions emphasized the same characteristics. Yet Merskey, in 1967, had already raised the question whether the guilt, resentment, hostility and transformation of affect and libido could occur without pain being present.

Most classical psychosomatic studies on the other hand give psychological portraits of different pain patient categories: the migrainous is described as conformist, dignified, sensitive and intelligent (10, 13); the lombalgic is an insecure, giving-up or frustrated individual (12). Tenseness and unexpressed unconscious aggressiveness such as obsessionality are usually invoked in tension headaches (13, 26). Moreover, several authors (16, 22) have stressed the existence of depressive and anxious features in patients complaining of pain, sometimes even accompanied by a risk of ego-disruption.

None of these features, however, are specific to pain patients. As early as 1973, the author wondered why anxiety or depression in some patients is expressed by pain rather than by any other type of psychological or physical expression. In other words, anxiety, depression, conflict, guilt, hostility (conscious or not), frustration and insecurity are present in many persons. Yet chronic pain is rare. Why then do only some people become chronic pain patients?

The characteristics we have just briefly summarized under the title "Classical Psychodynamic View of Pain Patients" are useful in individual case studies. However, they refer to nonspecific personality parameters. Thus, they are not enough for building a general model of how one becomes a pain patient.

PAIN-PRONENESS

In 1951 and 1959, Engel (6, 7) cast an original light on the problem. Going beyond the more classical description of the feelings and needs that the pain expressed, Engel referred more specifically to the development of the patients with punitive or abusing parents.

Suffering, in them, was learned in childhood. His patients presented with atypical facial pain. Engel considered them as presenting an hysterical conversion. However, reviewing their past, he emphasized the frequency of self-punitive behavior, including unnecessary surgery. Moreover, a pain

sion existed in conditions of misfortune or where there were other
es for suffering. Pain appeared thus to be learned as a way of feeling
an behaving very early in one's life. The early experience of pain sustained
the suffering role that these patients played. The concept of "pain-proneness" was born.

PAIN AS A WAY OF COMMUNICATION

Szasz (21) stated that pain refers to the perception of a threat to the
integrity of the body, however objective or imaginary. Yet pain is a way of
communication with others too. Pain can be a means of requesting help
from another person or a means of transmitting the idea of being unfairly
treated, abandoned, unloved or punished. Moreover, persisting pain can be
considered as an aggression against frustrating surroundings.

PAIN AS A NEUROVEGETATIVE VICIOUS CIRCLE

Another direction was explored by a surgeon, Leriche (11), who was
confronted with numerous intractable pain patients asking for surgical relief.
How many tremendous, unbearable pain states are still present years after
a slight common injury, such as a fall, a fracture, a simple prick! According
to Leriche, some persons experience as painful, sensations which for others
are simply disagreeable or eventually inconsequential.

He denied the validity of explaining this as fabrication or hysterical
conversion and invoked a neurovegetative conditioning of the sensation; the
peripheral vasomotor disturbances usually related to pain originating in
injuries would extend to cerebral blood circulation and would change
diencephalic expressions such as mood and character. His physiological
explanations can probably be considered as old-fashioned. However, the
concept of a distortion of the sensation leading to a feedback of vasomotor
and mood disturbances can be useful.

In the particular case of posttraumatic headaches, Brenner et al. (3)
referred to the hypothesis of a vicious circle: brain injury would provoke
affective changes, followed by vascular modification and secondary anxi-
ogenic headaches.

Contemporary versions of neurovegetative interactions invoke concepts
involving brain chemistry and endorphins, autonomic nervous system and
skeletal muscle reflex abnormalities.

CURRENT VIEWS ON PAIN PATIENTS

Much has been written more recently on pain and on pain control.
Different categories of pain patients, especially low-back sufferers (5), have
been carefully studied during the past years, with the help of personality
tests. Some studies can be considered as exemplary of a trend.

Sternbach et al. (20) examined 117 low-back pain patients seen consecu-
tively. They demonstrated that hypochondriasis, depression and hysteria

scores in the Minnesota Multiphasic Personality Inventory (M.M.P.I.) were significantly higher than normal in chronic pain patients whereas they remained within normal limits in patients with acute pain.

Bond (1) came to a different conclusion. He demonstrated the role of personality factors in relation to pain in 52 women with cancer of the cervix at the same clinical stage. Complaints of pain were shown to be associated primarily with extraversion, and lack of complaint was associated with introversion. Neuroticism scores were lower in patients without pain and higher in patients with pain. Bond considered as not sufficient the usual argument that pain increases emotionality. Referring to Eysenck's theory on emotionality, he argued that the susceptibility of an individual to increased emotionality—in other words, the neuroticism—could depend on a particular reactivity within the reticulolimbic system, predisposing to personality traits.

Fordyce (8) considers pain complaint as a behavior sensitive to environmental reinforcement. Pain occurring initially in response to nociception can remain as the result of conditioning.

Pain behavior is described by Fordyce as being a complex social communication involving all forms of behavior commonly understood to reflect the presence of nociception, including speech, facial expression, posture, seeking health care attention, taking medications, refusing to work. He demonstrated in a group of 77 chronic low-back pain patients that pain behavior diminished while exercising to tolerance, contrary to what was expected.

Merskey and Hester (15) clearly demonstrated that it was possible to relieve pain due to chronic lesions of the nervous system, including carcinomas, with a combination of phenothiazines, tricyclic antidepressant drugs and antihistaminics. The results were good even in cases wherein no emotional disturbances were apparent. This might be seen to support the concept of latent depression.

The interest of these studies lies not only in their results, with which they were able to support some of the assumptions that had been made in earlier clinical studies, but also in their methods.

Nevertheless, no single theory or work has given an adequate model of why some persons become chronic pain patients. However, putting together elements coming from different authors, we get some pieces of the puzzle, i.e., the conversion to pain of unconscious emotions, the presence of neuroticism and depression, a pain-proneness generated by punitive and abusive parents and linked with early suffering, the use of pain complaint as a way of communication, and neurovegetative and behavioral conditioning.

ANAMNESTIC STUDIES OF PAIN PATIENTS

With regard to attempting to construct a model, the author had studied extensively 63 cases of "intractable" pain of benign origin that had been referred to the neurosurgical department; she followed the evolution of 57 of these cases under various treatments, including psychotherapy (23). Except for two of them, all of the pain patients had already presented numerous medical problems prior to their current pain symptomatology (Table 3.1).

Another study (24) focused on the onset of facial pain in 13 cases of cluster headache and in 15 cases of atypical facial neuralgia. In recent research (25), 40 chronic pain patients attending an acupuncture consultation were compared with a control group of 50 chronic otorhinolaryngological patients. Former mental illnesses (mostly depression) were proven to be significantly more numerous in pain patients (Table 3.2). Also, depressions were significantly more numerous in pain patient's families than in the control group (Table 3.3). This frequent familial nervous imbalance could be one of the reasons that in the major proportion of the patients the childhood had been so poor, even miserable. The author has noted that most pain patients indeed had suffered from a severe early affective deprivation (23, 24).

Of 63 chronic intractable pain patients from the 1978 study (23), 40% had

TABLE 3.1. *Medical Antecedents (Violon, 1978)*
N = 63

	Number	%
Other pain syndromes	38	60
Depressions	25	39
Severe infection	25	39
Accidents	21	33

TABLE 3.2. *Former Mental Diseases (Violon and Giurgea, 1980)*

	Pain Patients		Control Patients	
	N	%	N	%
Presence	10	25	4	10
Absence	30	75	46	90

$X^2 = 4,88; P < 0.05.$

TABLE 3.3. *Depression in the Patient's Family (Violon and Giurgea, 1980)*

	Pain Patients		Control Patients	
	N	%	N	%
Presence	13	33	6	12
Absence	27	67	44	88

$X^2 = 5,6; P < 0.02.$

not lived their childhood with both parents and 23% had been abandoned. Moreover, 82% of the pain patients complained of a lack of affection during their childhood; in 63% of the cases an open rejection was manifested and in 19% the problem consisted of a lack of bodily demonstration of affection from excessively cold parents. Finally, 37% of the group had been battered children.

The author could not, however, significantly demonstrate again these findings about early affective deprivation in her last comparative study; this difference in the results seemed to be due to a difference in the methods of both studies. The first one indeed was founded upon anamnestic and therapeutic interviews, the second one upon questionnaires. Patients acknowledged in the interview what they denied when presented with a questionnaire that they must complete. Many seemed guided in the latter situation by a feeling of guilt, as if they were signing an accusation against their parents or substitute parents.

There has been one or several cases of chronic pain in the families of most pain patients (Table 3.4). This kind of "familial pain model" is far more frequent in pain patients than in other chronic patients without pain.

More than 60% of the patients, whatever their pain consisted of, were undoubtedly depressed before the onset of pain (Table 3.5). In some patients the depression was obvious, with suicidal tendencies; most of the time the depressions were masked ones and had not been diagnosed and treated.

Depression and pain are intimately linked. Depression has to be considered as a *determinant* of chronic pain and not simply as a consequence of it.

Forty percent of the patients assigned their pain to an emotional stress or

TABLE 3.4. *Chronic Pain in Patients' Families (Violon and Giurgea, 1980)*

| | Pain Patients | | Control Patients | |
	N	%	N	%
Presence	31	78	22	44
Absence	9	22	28	56

$X^2 = 10.3; P < 0.01.$

TABLE 3.5. *Depression Previous to the Onset of Pain*

| | (Violon, 1978) Pain Patients | | (Violon, 1980) | | | |
| | | | Cluster Headaches | | Atypical Facial Pains | |
	N	%	N	%	N	%
Presence	38	66	8	61	10	66
Absence or doubtful	19	34	5	39	5	34

TABLE 3.6. *The Precipitation of Pain (Violon, 1978)*

Bodily "Causes"		Emotional "Causes"	
Surgery	10	Emotional traumatism	20
Dental treatment	9	Depression	3
Medical treatment	1	Total	23
Injury	11		
Effort	2		40%
Cold	2		
Total	35		
		Not investigated	5
	60%		

a depression (Table 3.6). In 60% of the patients, pain began after some bodily event. However, even when the pain is ascribed to an initial somatic modification, a causal relationship often seems less probable than the constitution of an "organic spine"! Indeed, 56% of the patients who incriminated a bodily cause precipitating their pain were already depressed before the bodily event and subsequent onset of pain. Thus the sequence was in fact: depression–bodily modification–onset of pain.

THE PROCESS INVOLVED IN BECOMING A CHRONIC PAIN PATIENT: A PROPOSED MODEL

At this stage, we can make a further step in the integration of these different results and conceptions in order to build a proposed model of how one becomes a chronic pain patient (Fig. 3.1). The model is schematic of this whole dynamic process, but it is incomplete. Intrapsychic factors are accounted for in more detail, notwithstanding the importance of environmental, communication, and psychophysiological factors which are not expanded in the schema. The preferential narcissistic investment in the body rather than in fantasmic, relational and affective or intellectual life ought also to be taken into account. Moreover the lack of capacity to verbalize one's tensions and conflicts, usual in chronic pain and psychosomatic patients, ought to be stressed. Within certain limits, language and behavior can substitute for each other. The pain patient would "act" his psychic suffering rather than expressing it verbally. Nevertheless, this model can perhaps offer a support to the conceptualization of the different views and treatments concerning chronic pain patients.

Failure of Medical and Psychiatric Formulations

THE CONCEPT OF SYMPTOMATIC PAIN

"Pain Equals Disease"

For the patient, persisting pain is a frightening experience, often more so than the disease in itself. In a study comparing 103 patients with chronic

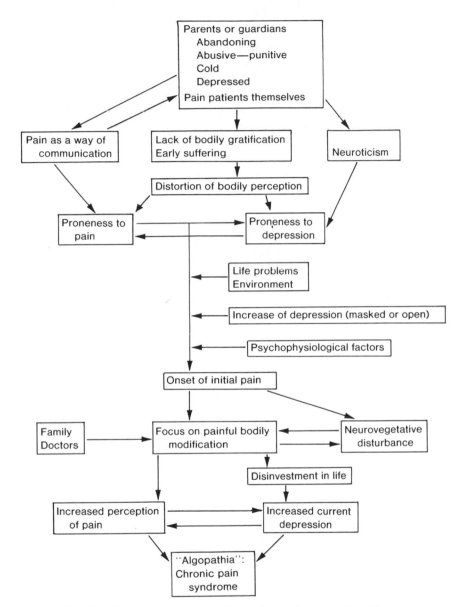

Fig. 3.1. Process involved in becoming a chronic pain patient.

benign pain with 22 cancer pain patients, Silbret and Rosomoff (18) reported an approximate 100% increase in depression in both groups. The benign pain group, however, reported more suicidal ideation and more feeling of rejection and abandonment than did the cancer group.

Chronic benign pain patients indeed experience a particularly difficult situation in their relationship with doctors. For the physician, pain is a clue to a more or less hidden disease which he has to uncover. The traditional model of pain is linked to the concept of objective causality. The first equation mentioned above assimilates pain to the visible surface of the hidden iceberg-disease. The conscientious classical physician has thus to discover the supposedly simple, precise, clear-cut cause of the supposedly symptomatic pain. Repeated and various examinations are practiced, leading possibly to surgical acts. Leriche (11) has described this process in some cases of posttraumatic intractable pain, phantom limbs and painful stumps for instance: amputations, reamputations, nerve section neurectomies, alcohol blocks, repeated searches for neuromas, sympathectomies, cordotomies . . . ; 10, 20 and even 40 operations . . . and the pain reappearing each time. Not all cases are so dramatic, but the same way of thinking usually leads to the same maneuvers.

Brihaye and I (4) have observed such a case. It is worth relating here.

R.B. was a 48-year-old worker, sent to our department with the diagnosis of causalgia. His medical anamnesis was as follows:

27.2.68:	Work accident. Left forefinger wounded by a particle of iron
28.2.68:	Partial extraction of this small piece
4, 12 and 19.3.68:	New unsuccessful attempts to extract the particle
2.4.68:	Successful extraction; good healing but the scar remains sensitive
28.5.68:	Electrocoagulation of the scar
25.6.68:	Idem—amelioration of the abnormal sensitivity
January 1969:	Aggravation of the sensitivity
13.1.69:	Excision—curettage
28.1.69:	Electrocoagulation
5.3.69:	Excision of the scarred area of the forefinger and grafting; pain remains
9.4.69:	New resection; larger grafting; normal cicatrization but remaining hyperesthesia around the grafting
1.7.69:	Local injection of cortisone; no relief
August 1969:	Aggravated hyperesthesia. The patient describes a pain compared to a sensation of tearing of the flesh around the area of the grafting. He feels a distention in his finger. Touching with it is unpleasant. A trial of treatment with meprobamate-promethazine does not relieve the pain.
October 1969:	Aggravation. Pain extends to the three fingerjoints. Clear-cut trophic disturbances are marked: paleness, coldness, thinning down of the finger, severe demineralization of the forefinger observed with radiography.
Nov/Dec. 1969:	Unsuccessful local injections
February 1970:	Status quo of pain at the forefinger; emergence of intermittent pain at the forearm, the internal aspect of the arm and the left shoulder

20.2.70:   Infiltration of the left stellate ganglion with Xylocaine followed by temporary relief

3.3.70:   Thoracotomy in the third space, sympathectomy of the inferior part of the stellate ganglion and of the ganglions Th 2–Th 3. The aspect of the forefinger becomes normal again; hyperesthesia disappears on the first and second joint but remains unchanged at the third fingerjoint.

15.4.70:   Surgical resection of the third fingerjoint, including the extremity of the second one: disappearance of the pain

Beginning of June 1970: Resurgence of the pain at the top of the stump, in the vicinity of the scar

17.6.70:   Useless local injection of alcohol

26.6.70:   Surgical resection of the second forefinger and of the top of the first one. Pain disappears.

25.8.70:   Resurgence of the hyperesthesia of the stump and of the scar; hyperesthesia appears also in the area of the scar of thoracotomy.

1.9.70:   Useless injections of Xylocaine

September–October 1970: Useless treatment with trifluperidol first, then with flupenthixol and melitracen

In 1971, the patient was sent to our department and treated successfully with a multidisciplinary therapy including psychotherapy, thymoanaleptic, anxiolytic and neuroleptic medication and massages. He became able to work again. He is still (1981) followed up once a year.

Another of our cases is demonstrative.

At the age of 42, A.S. began to feel pain in the area of the third division of the trigeminal nerve, on the right hemiface. Consisting initially of acute episodes, the pain evolved notwithstanding a treatment with tegretol and became constant. The patient underwent a surgical section of the third branch of the trigeminal nerve. Pain disappeared for 3 weeks, then it came back, covering the whole right hemiface and the right neck: violent, continuous, burning. The lips burned, photophobia developed, mastication was difficult. Multiple tooth extractions were done without relieving the pain. A trigeminal tractotomy at the bulbar level proved useless; pain reappeared 3 days after the operation. A psychotropic and psychotherapeutic treatment conducted in our department relieved the patient. However, pain reappeared when the patient went back to her usual lonely life.

Not all chronic pain cases are so dramatic but the same type of classical medical thinking in terms of direct causality often leads to the same erroneous maneuvers. Moreover, the patient's insistence on relief sometimes induces an inappropriate medical or surgical response in the doctors, by provoking in them feelings such as pity, anger, impotence, or personal overpotency contrasting with their colleagues' failures.

One of the more recent cases we have treated in our clinic is a good demonstration of a doctor's inappropriate reaction.

R.G., a 43-year-old farmer, underwent a work accident 9 years ago, with an open head injury and a tearing out of the brachial plexus. Only a few nerves were preserved, which still allowed him slight movements of his arm and elbow. The sensibility of the arm, hand and fingers was completely lost. The patient began to suffer from phantom pains in his still present limb.

A surgeon performed an alcohol block of the remaining nerves of the plexus. Following that, the patient lost completely the motor function of this arm and the pain increased severely, the depression too. We could only partially relieve it, using transcutaneous electrical nerve stimulation along with antidepressants.

"No Disease Equals No Pain"

The search for a determinate organic origin of persistent pain sometimes succeeds.

For instance, one of the most recent cases we had the opportunity to treat was a 43-year-old woman with low-back and leg pains that had lasted for 2 years. She had seen several doctors and been diagnosed as neurotic: she was indeed. No motor or sensory deficit accompanied the pain. She had an emotionally disturbed past and present life. However, she was found to have a triple lumbar disc herniation.

Most of the time, on the other hand, this research is unfruitful. How frustrating it is for the physician to be confronted by a complaining patient whose pain remains. Some doctors' reactions are aggressive. 'What the individual feels can be denied.' 'There are no reasons for the patient to complain of pain or even to feel pain as long as no physical disturbance is evident.'

The same reactions occur when a disease is considered as completely cured.

One of our 31-year-old female patients had had an accident 10 years before, with a traumatic lesion of the right knee followed by nine operations. The first one was for the lesion itself: the other ones, including a right lumbar sympathectomy, were for a persisting pain. According to some surgeons, the persistent pain indicated a remaining lesion, thus an indication for surgery. Others were derogatory about her mental health. One was frankly hostile and denied the patient's pain.

As the above vignettes demonstrate, the chronic pain patient may be treated as a malingerer, as mentally disturbed or as an hysteric.

"Pain Plus No Disease Equals Psychic Disturbance"

Most of the time, physicians do not lose their tempers and do not treat the patient with hostility. However, in the classical medical model of pain, if nothing is wrong in the soma, something must be wrong in the psyche. Patients' interminable journey from one surgeon to another and from one physiotherapist to the neurologist will probably also include a short stopover in the psychiatrist's or the psychologist's office.

"No Psychological Abnormality Equals No Explanation of Pain"

Then again the equation is erroneous. As Sternbach (19) observed, "The head-shrinker will do his best to soothe the patient's feelings and will try to determine whether the patient is crazy or a drug addict, or if the pain is 'psychosomatic.' These will all prove not to be the case, and this consultant will leave with few helpful recommendations."

Pinsky (17) underlined the pain patient's reluctance, disappointment, or even desperation when sent to the psychiatrist: the "real" doctors do not believe him, don't want to treat him any more, think that he exaggerates his pain, and consider him as crazy. For the pain patient, talking about his past, childhood, parents, family, or feelings makes no sense. He thinks he is receiving an inappropriate response to the question of his bodily pain since his psychic life is perceived as having nothing to do with his pain. The patient knows that his pain is not "imaginary" and feels misunderstood and rejected. Most psychiatrists and psychologists do not know about chronic pain patients. Consequently, their diagnosis too is clear-cut; 'normal or abnormal,' 'neurotic or not,' absence or presence of relevant personal problems able to explain the "conversion" or the "complaint." Sometimes they are reluctant to see these unusual cases. Classical psychiatrists do not cure chronic pain.

From the initial misunderstanding, the discomfort extends: the patient, the physician, the psychiatrist, the family too become involved. Trying to clarify this misunderstanding, we come again to the idea of objective causality. The cause of pain is supposed to be unidimensional: a simple identifiable (physical or mental) disease, injury or bodily dysfunction. (This is true not only for patients but for most doctors too.) Their long search for some relief is usually a search for the doctor who will be able to identify and take away the cause of their pain, and not just the pain in itself.

Naming the Pain: "Algopathia; Algopathic Patients"

Considering pain as a "real disease" in itself appears the only appropriate conceptual position for the doctors, and even more so for the patients and acquaintances. This position could avoid repeated useless and noxious investigations of a hypothetical lesional cause for pain, supposed by patients and physicians to be symptomatic of a disease. At this stage, an absolute necessity emerges: naming this trouble, as one would a disease.

The pain patient certainly needs to have a name and an explanation for what he feels as a painful illness. He needs it for himself in order to be able to comprehend what is going on in him. He needs it too for facing his environment and the questions about what is wrong with him. If no appropriate name is available, the patient is in a quandary: "I have a pain but the doctors say that nothing is wrong. So what then? Must I be considered as a mentally sick person?"

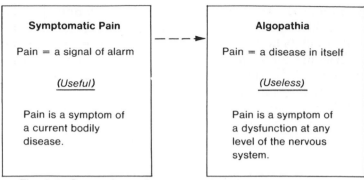

Fig. 3.2. Comparison of symptomatic pain and algopathia.

Even though psychological factors are generally definable in chronic pain, pain patients cannot be considered simply psychiatric. This alternative comes from a classical, however inacceptable, dichotomy: "the pain or disease is either a mental one or a bodily one," as if body and mind were two separate worlds functioning as parallels. We refuse this dichotomy as unrealistic and leading to no adequate treatment. This question of the mind-body dichotomy is dealt with in Chapter 2 by Prof. Merskey. The only reasonable position must be based on a principle of interaction between bodily perception, emotion and cognition.

Accordingly, we propose the term "*algopathia*" for chronic pain states which are not symptomatic of a current disease. "Algopathia" would thus be defined as "Any chronic pain not symptomatic of a current disease, that expresses either directly or through vascular or muscular painful modifications a dysfunction at any level of the nervous system."

Algopathia involves persistent or recurrent pain states whatever precipitated them (emotion, trauma, medical care, surgery or unknown factors) and would be discriminated from symptomatic pain, the existence of which is of course obvious and useful (Fig. 3.2).

Symptomatic pain usually has a vital utility. Algopathia has none and is even noxious. Algopathia must be treated as a distinct disorder, whereas the relief of symptomatic pain depends first on the treatment of the underlying causal disease.

In some cases, symptomatic pain can transform into algopathia; these are cases wherein pain remains when its cause has apparently been cured.

The Patient's Interminable Journey through the Medical Mill

During the interminable journey through the medical mill, the pain is still present, severe or torturing. Moreover, the patient feels lost, more anxious, or frankly desperate. The more anxious or depressed he becomes, the more violently he feels the pain. Progressively, he loses his status as an independent human being and becomes an object of care, sent from one practitioner to another, being palpated, pricked, radiographed, submitted to a variety of technical examinations, to innocuous or painful diagnostic means, and varied therapeutics, but less often carefully listened to and understood. His health can be compromised and his pain can be aggravated by multiplied inappropriate measures. Sternbach (19) has described the patients' successive hopefulness and disappointment and their progressively increased bitterness and resentment toward the doctors. Also the more the patient focuses his mind on his own body, the more he is invaded by the secret conviction of having a dangerous disease that no doctor is able to find and to cure or that the physicians are hiding from him.

Although not openly expressed, the fear of having an occult disease such as a cancer is usually present in patients with a chronic pain. Bodily sensations become even more distorted as time passes, with pain occupying more and more of the patient's consciousness. In some patients, this process develops immediately or quickly after a painful injury, operation or disease. This is reminiscent of the vicious circle described by Leriche (11) 30 years ago, according to which pain in some individuals does not disappear normally with its initial cause but remains and increases.

As the investment in bodily symptoms increases, the interest in professional, social and personal life decreases. The patient is often absent from his job because of his pain and his medical consultations and may cease work altogether. The housekeeper forsakes her housework. The patient loses interest in children and friends, or their presence becomes unbearable. He or she becomes isolated with his or her companion, the pain.

The pain complaint can, however, have an apparent positive effect on family cohesion. Particular attention may be devoted to the pain patient, who is asked repeated questions about the pain and about his bodily sensations. He is treated as a sick person who has to be particularly spared. This treatment can reinforce the anxious focusing on the body and can comfort the patient in his sick role through secondary gain.

Thus, either rejection or attentive care can increase pain perception in the patients. The pain patient's journey from one consultation to the other resembles what is often called in French, "la quête du Graal," an interminable, desperate and finally useless quest. The patient is no more a subject, a responsible and independent person, but becomes an object in the hands of the doctors. Here again, depression is in the foreground (Table 3.7) (23, 24).

The patient becomes confused. As time passes, he understands less and less his own situation. When feeling pain, everybody has in mind the example of toothache, where the normal evolution is for pain to disappear when the bad tooth is extracted. In a situation of persistence or aggravation of the pain, the pain patient does not understand that his own personality

TABLE 3.7. *Current Depression*

	(Violon, 1978) Pain Patients		(Violon, 1980) Cluster Headaches		Atypical Facial Pains	
	N	%	N	%	N	%
Presence	53	85	11	84	15	100
Absence or doubtful	9	15	2	16	—	—

has some relationship with his disease. He remains attached to the concept of bodily damage. Becoming desperate, he may consult charlatans and healers.

If he does not have the chance to be treated in a pain clinic, he often will become an invalid, sapped by his pain, shrinking his life and world, remaining in chair or bed, and maybe eventually ending his life.

REFERENCES

1. BOND, M. R. Pain and personality in cancer patients. In *Advances in Pain Research and Therapy, Vol. 1.* edited by J. J. Bonica and D. Albe-Fessard, Raven Press, New York, 1976.
2. BOURHIS, A. AND SPITALIER, J. M. La douleur-maladie en carcinologie. *Biol. Med., 59:* 427–458, 1970.
3. BRENNER, C., FRIEDMAN, A. P. AND CARTER, S. Psychological factors in the etiology and treatment of chronic headache. *Psychosom. Med., 11:* 53–56, 1949.
4. BRIHAYE, J., AND VIOLON, A. La douleur causalgique. *Acta Chir. Belg., 3:* 195–200, 1978.
5. CUMMINGS, C., EVANSKI, P. M., DEBENEDETTI, M. J., ANDERSON, E. E., AND WAUGH, T. R. Use of MMPI to predict outcome of treatment for chronic pain. In *Advances in Pain Research and Therapy, Vol. 3,* edited by J. J. Bonica, J. C. Liebeskind, and D. G. Albe-Fessard. Raven Press, New York, 1979.
6. Engel, G. L. Primary atypical facial neuralgia: An hysterical conversion symptom. *Psychosom. Med., 13:* 375–396, 1951.
7. ENGEL, G. "Psychogenic" pain and the pain-prone patient. *Am. J. Med., 26:* 899–918, 1959.
8. FORDYCE, W. E. Environmental factors in the genesis of low back pain. In *Advances in Pain Research and Therapy, Vol. 3.* edited by J. J. Bonica, J. C. Liebeskind, and D. G. Albe-Fessard, Raven Press, New York, 1979.
9. HEIMANN H., BOBON-SCHROD, H., SCHMOCKER, A. M., AND BOBON, D. P. Autoévaluation de l'humeur par une liste d'adjectifs, la "Befindlichkeits-Skala" (BS) de Zerssen. *L'Encephale, I:* 165–183, 1975.
10. KNOPF, O. Preliminary report on personality studies in thirty migraine patients. *J. Nerv. Ment. Dis., 82:* 270–285, 400–414, 1935 a and b.
11. LERICHE, R. *La Chirurgie de la Douleur.* Masson et Cie, Paris VIe, 1949.
12. LUBAN-PLOZZA, B. AND POLDINGER, W. *Le Malade Psychosomatique et le Medecin Praticien.* Ed. Roche, Bâle., 1974.
13. LUMINET, D. Les céphalées: Traité de psychologie médicale 3. *IV:* 133–143, 1973.
14. MELZACK, R. *The Puzzle of Pain: Penguin Science of Behaviour.* Harmondsworth, Middlesex, England, 1973.
15. MERSKEY, H., AND HESTER, R. N. The treatment of chronic pain with psychotropic drugs. *Postgrad. Med. J., 48:* 594–598, 1972.
16. MERSKEY, H., AND SPEAR, F. G. *Pain: Psychological and Psychiatric Aspects.* Baillière, Tindall and Cassell, London, 1967.

17. PINSKY, J. J. Psychodynamics and psychotherapy in the treatment of patients with chronic intractable pain. In *Pain: Research and Treatment*, edited by B. L. J. Crue. Academic Press, New York, San Francisco, London, 1975.
18. SILBRET, M., AND ROSOMOFF, H. *Psychological Characteristics of Pain Patients with Benign and Malignant Disease. Pain Abstracts, Vol. 1.* I.A.S.P., Seattle, 1978.
19. STERNBACH, R. A. *Pain Patients. Traits and Treatment.* Academic Press, New York, San Francisco, London, 1974.
20. STERNBACH, R. A., WOLF, S. R., MURPHY, R. W., AND AKESON, W. H. Traits of pain patients: The low-back "loser." *Psychosomatics, 14:* 226–229, 1973.
21. SZASZ, T. *Pain and Pleasure: A Study of Bodily Feelings.* Basic Books, New York, 1957.
22. VIOLON, A. Pain as a disease: Psychological investigation. *Headache, 13(1):* 25–28, 1973.
23. VIOLON, A. *Le syndrome douloureux chronique: Étude psychologique.* Ph.D. Thesis, Brussels University, 1978.
24. VIOLON, A. The onset of facial pain. *Psychother. Psychosom., 34:* 11–16, 1980.
25. VIOLON, A., AND GIURGEA, D. Psychological and psychosocial characteristics of pain patients (manuscript in preparation). 1980.
26. WOLFF, H. G., AND WOLF, S. *Headaches: Their Nature and Treatment.* Little, Brown & Co., Boston, 1953.

4

The Sick-Role and Chronic Pain

EUGENE B. GALLAGHER, Ph.D.
SYLVIA WROBEL, M.A.

A major contribution of medical sociology to the understanding of illness in society is the concept of the sick-role. Formulated by the late sociological theorist Talcott Parsons, the sick-role concept codifies the various privileges and responsibilities which attach to the role of a sick person in our society.

In part one of this chapter we summarize the sick-role, presenting its four analytic components. Next, we consider the particular modifications in the sick-role concept which are warranted by the situation of the person suffering from a chronic illness. This establishes a basis for sociological examination of the role of the chronic pain patient. Although both bear a chronic affliction, the pain patient who suffers severe headaches, neuralgia, or low backaches is in a different position from the patient with a diagnosable medical condition such as diabetes. The invisible, subjective nature of pain has many implications for the pain patient's relationships within his family and social groups, for his interactions with health professionals, and for his conception of himself. We further develop the view that success in dealing with the pain patient, as with other chronic illness patients, must be measured by the extent to which the patient is able, with professional guidance, to effect an adaptive balance between the constraints of his affliction and the claims and opportunities of his life-situation.

Chronic pain has recently become the focus of new theoretical explanations, professional roles, and treatment programs. The interdisciplinary pain clinic has emerged as a major institutional modality. Part two of this chapter deals with these developments and pays particular attention to their significance within the context of academic medicine and in relation to prevailing assumptions about the doctor-patient relationship.

Part three briefly examines chronic pain treatment in the light of other developments in contemporary medicine. We suggest that, with the increasing burden of chronic disease in society, treatment must be supplemented by rehabilitative approaches in clinical settings which integrate diverse specialties and foster new role-definitions for both patients and staff.

The Sick-Role Applied to Chronic Illness and Pain

In Parsons' original formulation of the sick-role, there are four components (7). Two are rights or claims that the sick person can make legitimately upon the behavior and feelings of others. Two are obligations and responsibilities of the sick person, that is, claims which society can make legitimately upon him or her.

First, the sick-role occupant is not held responsible for his or her condition and is spared blame or censure for being ill. Illness is viewed as involuntary, not the victim's fault. A person may suffer an accident through recklessness, carelessly expose himself to infection or maintain a health-risking way of life through heavy smoking, overeating, or working in a toxic environment. But any illness or medical condition that results is regarded as the expression of natural forces which, although their pathological mechanisms may be understood scientifically and the contribution of the individual to his or her own increased susceptibility be fully recognized, nonetheless are considered beyond the control of the individual. The person who is struck by disease or accident is not only shielded from blame but is entitled to sympathy and support, depending upon the severity of his condition and the degree of suffering it causes him.

Second, the person admitted to the sick-role is exempted from his usual obligations, whether they be social, family, school or work. An exemption may be as trivial as allowing the person who has a sore throat to whisper and to refrain from the greetings and small talk customary in social intercourse. It may be as major as release from all responsibilities for going to work and earning a living for one's family and self. Depending on the severity of the sickness, the sick-role takes various degrees of precedence over other role responsibilities and obligations.

How an exemption becomes socially recognized and accepted is an important question. Minor exemptions are sanctioned through informal social understandings, as when someone with a cold is urged to leave work and take care of himself by going home to bed. In instances involving lawsuits, employment sick leaves, or disability claims, exemption may require a more formal statement from the physician, who is the usual gatekeeper to the sick-role and who must validate the claims of the sick person. Validation may also be sought in order to win sympathy and support from family members who do not take one's illness very seriously and who may be reluctant to allow one of their members to lay aside, even temporarily, customary responsibilities within the household. This has important implications for the patient with chronic pain.

The third analytic component of the sick-role sets forth the obligation of the sick-role occupant to think and act as if his sickness were an undesirable state, to be cured if possible, otherwise to be minimized or managed as effectively as possible. On the one hand, he is spared blame for his condition and may be granted various exemptions from responsibility and various other compensations. On the other hand, he is urged to rid himself of the condition; he should not find the exemptions and compensations so enticing that he begins to regard the sickness with which they are associated as somewhat desirable. To speak of the sick-role, rather than merely a state of sickness, suggests precisely that the sick person becomes the focus of social expectations. These expectations tend to shore up the sick person's potentially faltering motivations toward recovery and the resumption of normal roles.

In this generalized attitudinal obligation of the sick-role, one most clearly sees illness from the sociological perspective of deviance. In sociological theory, deviance is behavior that departs from the moral expectations of society. Crime is a familiar example of deviant behavior. Illness can also be seen as deviance. It threatens the continued smooth functioning of society because it limits the ability of its bearers, the sick, to carry out their normal social roles. At the same time, the sick burden society with their need for treatment and special consideration. The stance toward the sick might well have been neglect or disapproval rather than sympathy. (This idea is dealt with in a novel by Samuel Butler—*Erewhon*—the story of a mythical land where the social deviancies of illness and criminality are interchanged.)

The sick-role is a specific social creation which thwarts such tendencies and which enhances the opportunity of the sick person to recover from, or adapt to, his illness. Traces of antagonism toward the sick do at times show through the social fabric, as when a sick person is suspected of malingering or of finding sympathy and attention too enjoyable. The psychiatric concept of "secondary gain" has application to physical illness. The fact society lauds individuals such as Albert Schweitzer and Mother Teresa of Calcutta, who make an extraordinary commitment to the care of the sick, indicates that the more mundane expectations which fall upon most persons in dealing with the sick do require a level of personal investment and concern which cannot be taken for granted. The supportive, noncensorious posture which others adopt toward the sick person is a seemingly natural sentiment, but this sentiment has a fund of social energy and patterning behind it, expressed sociologically in the sick-role concept.

The fourth component states that the sick-role occupant is obligated to seek appropriate help in dealing with his illness. This follows logically from the previous components. If the sickness is not the person's "fault," could he be expected to cure it by an act of will? If he is exempted from other role responsibilities in the expectation that he will try to return to them as soon as possible, then it is incumbent upon him to find a means of cure or improvement. We have seen that the greater the severity of the sickness, the greater is the exemption from ordinary role responsibilities. Likewise here, the greater the severity of the sickness, the greater is the obligation to seek appropriate help.

In modern societies, the medical profession, with its associated roles and institutions, is the conventional help-source (although nonmedical sources such as chiropractic and faith-healing are also available and find favor among particular social strata and subcultures). In obtaining medical care, the sick person becomes a patient and thereby enters into a system of social expectations which extend and intensify those expectations associated with the sick-role. He is placed in contact with health personnel whose professionally stabilized motivations and attitudes have a higher degree of integration and objectivity than do the affectively toned motivations and attitudes of friends and relatives. The physician is expected not only to provide competent technical service in the form of diagnosis and treatment but also to provide support and encouragement toward the patient's recovery or other most favorable outcome.

If we had to resolve the sick-role into a single master component, combining the above four components, we might say that it consists of a *socially legitimized dependency*.

That the sick-role confers a dependent status upon its bearer is seen clearly enough in the notion of exemption from one's normal responsibilities and duties. It is important to note, however, that sick-role dependency is not the more nearly total and permanent dependency of a mentally retarded, or physically disabled, or infirm elderly person but rather is a qualified dependency. Although much of the sick person's dependency is due to the sickness itself, he is expected to shed as much of it as he can, to seek and cooperate with appropriate sources of health care, and to strive toward recovery. The socially-legitimized, or bestowed, dependency can be seen as a benefit conditionally allowed in exchange for the sick person's doing what he can to improve his lot.

THE SICK-ROLE IN CHRONIC ILLNESS

There is substantial agreement among medical sociologists that Parsons' formulation of the sick-role captures and distills the essential elements of the social meaning of much illness in our society. It is too generalized, however, to portray adequately all categories of illness. With reference to the familiar acute/chronic illness distinction, the sick-role concept as presented above fits acute illness better than chronic illness. Additional elements must be incorporated to cover the person with a chronic illness.

Unlike acute problems such as most infectious diseases and broken bones, chronic diseases are long-term and ongoing, often with little likelihood of cure. Once given, social support and exemptions are likely to be equally long-term, possibly permanent, although they may wax and wane as the condition fluctuates. In many cases, the person with a chronic illness is constrained and disabled in some directions but nonetheless can manage many ordinary responsibilities and he is established on a maintenance medical regimen, not requiring critical attention. His sick-role does not always diminish other roles.

Some chronic illnesses are subject to episodic fluctuations, such as an asthma attack or diabetic coma. The person temporarily enters an encompassing acute sick-role until the condition is under the normal level of control. Then he resumes the ongoing chronic sick-role. Otherwise this less dominant chronic sick-role may be of variable import and obviousness to different members of the person's circle of family and friends. It may be of major import to the spouse of a heart attack victim who is limited in his household and sexual capability, while it may not even be perceived by his business associates.

In a review of the sick-role concept, Gallagher (5) advanced the notion that, in the chronic sick-role, adaptation rather than cure is the most favorable outcome for the patient. In a general biological sense, adaptation conveys the idea of best fit between an organism and its environment. For the chronically ill or disabled person, adaptation means reciprocal adjustment between person and sociophysical setting. The intensively organized medical environment is appropriate for acute illness; what is necessary for the chronically ill person is some degree of environmental protection and support, appropriately related to the person's incapacities.

In the chronic patient's activities and mode of life, we see a second distinctive feature of the chronic sick-role. As compared with an acute sick-role, there is increased autonomy and responsibility for maintenance of health within the chronic sick-role. The role-occupant's responsibility is to maintain the highest possible level of health and functioning–not complicate his illness or lose ground needlessly. His activities must be consistent with medical judgment, but, since his activities occur outside the sphere of intensive acute medical care, the chronically ill person's life will embrace values and functions other than sheer compliance with medical goals and procedures.

In summary, the chronic sick-role differs from the acute sick-role as follows: the chronic sick-role does not necessarily take precedence over other social roles. The role-occupant does not even require recognition of his role by all role partners. To a greater extent than the person in the acute sick-role, he is an autonomous agent in society, being dominated by the claims of neither illness nor medical treatment. He cannot, however, be considered to have all the resources of a healthy person to commit to endeavors; some exemptions may be necessary to accomodate his impairment or limitations.

THE CHRONIC PAIN PATIENT

Pain is a common and highly significant element in one's self-definition as being sick and in one's consequent entry into the sick-role. Sudden, acute pain serves as an almost unqualified immediate pathway into the sick-role, taking precedence over any other bodily awareness or self-interpretation. Everything comes to a halt in the face of sudden, acute pain. The afflicted person has full social permission to seek relief, and medicine has evolved anesthetic techniques which serve effectively to tide sufferers over short periods of intense pain. The chronic pain of rheumatoid arthritis, migraine headaches, and the low back syndrome presents a different situation, clinically and socially. Pain relief measures which can be used in emergencies or occasionally for brief periods cannot be used indefinitely because they may addict or otherwise incapacitate the patient. Also, the chronic pain patient usually has, despite his suffering, many unimpaired capacities which he may not want to surrender to the process of obtaining relief.

In chronic pain, it is important to distinguish between pain as a symptom of something else and pain itself as the major, or only, medical problem— that is, pain as a clinical category. When pain is a symptom of definite disease or medical condition, it is desirable to treat the underlying cause; curing the disease usually results in the abolition of the pain, along with other symptoms. In chronic diseases, the diminution or abolition of accompanying pain is one measure of how far a chronic condition has been brought under control. Further, when pain accompanies a disease, it can then be correlated with an observable lesion or other manifestation of the disease.

Pain itself is a subjective experience that cannot be measured objectively but is socially shared in the sense that all of us recognize instinctively its manifestations—the doubling over, the hand to the afflicted part—and we often have some expectation as to how much something "should" hurt. Medical personnel have explicitly developed expectations concerning painful conditions which they see frequently—expectations as to both the intensity and the duration of the pain, what Fagerhaugh and Strauss call the "pain trajectory" (2). Deviations from this expected trajectory are the basis for efforts to pull the patient back into line with expectations, whether it be urging patients to express more pain or ask for more pain medication or, in the case of someone expressing more pain than seems "reasonable," dismissing the patient's complaints and withholding requested medication.

In the traditional medical view, pain can be placed along a polar continuum between "organic" and "psychic" processes. As a purely subjective phenomenon, dependent upon the patient's report and related to his emotional state, personality, and life-experience, pain is seen to lie far toward the psychic pole. Modern medicine has a strong bias toward the objective assessment of disease and the quantification of its pathological mechanisms. It thus prefers to deal with phenomena on the organic side of the continuum. Objective medical diagnosis of organic conditions frequently can account for pain and other subjective complaints. With biomedical advances, it is becoming increasingly possible and important to fractionate out that portion of a patient's symptoms which may be due to organic causes from that portion which is psychically influenced—as for example in distinguishing specific brain deficit from the diffuse effects of the aging process and in determining how much of a child's behavior disorder can be attributed to determinate brain damage. Within the framework of modern organic medicine, it is difficult to deal with purely psychic processes, such as the chronic pain patient frequently presents.

For the amputee with phantom limb pain or the person with intractable lower back pain, there is no way to separate out the more objective organic part of the disease from the patient's experience of it. Frequently, the existence of pain can be determined *only* on the patient's own account, with no organic or objective evidence to parallel the patient's report. In cases in which an identifiable lesion does exist, providing a medical buttress for the patient's report, the correlation may not be high between severity of the patient's reported pain and the extent of somatic damage. An extreme point in the lack of correlation is represented in Henry K. Beecher's famous observation that soldiers wounded in battle often feel no pain: various psychological explanations, which themselves move in very different directions, can account for this (1). One soldier who is personally committed to battle and victory may be "distracted" out of pain by his desire to fight (as frenzied football players may not notice their broken ankle until it gives way under them as they try to return to the field), while another may experience his wound less as a source of pain than as a welcome release from further combat.

Although the role of the chronic pain patient falls within the general scope of the sick-role as it applies to chronically ill persons, the chronic pain role nevertheless constitutes a particular version of it. Because of the subjective nature of his complaint, the chronic pain patient is much more likely to have difficulty entering the sick-role and his perch there is far more fragile than that of persons with recognized diseases.

The majority of chronic pain patients have considered themselves sick for long periods. It is also characteristic of such patients that they will have undergone numerous medical consultations and procedures in an attempt to have their condition diagnosed, much less treated. Many have passed through a series of physicians and have even undergone surgery for pain relief, until they have exhausted traditional resources with no lasting help, a frustration to the physician as well as the patient.

Recent Institutional Programs and Concepts in Pain Treatment

At the same time, pain has been reconceptualized as a clinical problem in itself. Rather than pain being simply a symptom, the elusiveness of pain and the complex nature of chronic pain have stimulated a growing body of literature and theory. Furthermore, the failure of earlier treatment regimens to resolve the problems of many chronic pain patients has brought about new techniques. These include advances in neurosurgery and anesthesiology, the development of analgesic and tranquilizing drugs, the use of biofeedback equipment to measure physiological responses and to teach the patient how to exert some control over aspects of the autonomous nervous system, behavioral strategies such as behavior modification, and measures to objectify pain either semantically or by comparative readings of pain threshold/average pain/tolerance for individual patients.

The major institutional approach to chronic pain, consolidating the various new techniques, has been the creation of pain clinics, which explicitly categorize and deal with the chronic pain patient. The establishment of pain clinics and the categorization of pain patients exemplifies the process of medicalization, a broad social dynamic whereby many kinds of human distress formerly thought of as inscrutable, sufferable aspects of the human condition have come to be regarded as problems which can be rationally analyzed and potentially solved within a medical framework (3, 4). Mental disorder, obesity, dental malocclusion, criminal and delinquent behavior, juvenile hyperactivity, alcoholism, drug addiction, excess fertility or infertility, malnutrition, environmental health hazards, and even the natural process of aging have all been transformed from domains of human behavior which simply "happen" or are viewed as the proper concern of nonmedical experts such as judges, priests, or sages. They have been medicalized, or colonized, as legitimate concerns of the medical profession.

As a subject of medical concern, pain occupies a rather different position from the foregoing subjects, because pain relief has long been a very important item on medical agenda. The recent and growing focus on chronic pain can be seen as an "internal colonization" or the transformation of a traditional area of medical practice rather than as the grasping of a nonmedical concern, such as delinquent behavior, into the realm of medicine. Other examples of internal colonization can be seen in the contemporary handling of childbirth and operative anesthesia, which have been thoroughly medicalized through the medical specialties of obstetrics and anesthesiology.

Although pain relief measures are undertaken in virtually every site where medicine is practiced—whether private physician's office, hospital clinic, or group practice—pain clinics are found primarily in academic medical centers and teaching hospitals. Here are evolved approaches and techniques which may eventually diffuse into rank-and-file practice but which owe their origination to the depth and diversity of medical specialty resources, the urge to innovation which permeates academic medicine, and the clinical necessity imposed by referral of difficult cases to medical centers.

Unsolved problems not infrequently tend to generate multidisciplinary efforts to grapple with them. Pain clinics are multidisciplinary in composition, with diverse staffing patterns and eclectic treatment approaches. Since the general thrust of academic medicine is toward greater specialization and refinement within the various branches of medicine, the establishment of multidisciplinary pain clinics expresses an integrative thrust in the face of a general trend in the opposite direction. At present the clinics' institutional viability is closely linked to the entrepreneurial energy and academic-medical vision of the "first generation" of founders. In addition to professional leadership, there is a matrix of intellectual resources which define the nature of the medical problem and appropriate strategies for dealing with it. An approximate sketch of this matrix is as follows.

The key personnel in pain clinics are drawn, in many instances, from both sides of the organic-psychic dichotomy—a psychologist or psychiatrist representing the psychic side, and a neurologist or internist representing the organic side. In identifying staff with opposite sides of this dichotomy, we do not suggest that they have a mutually confrontational, ideologically polarized concept of the essential nature or treatment of pain, such as psychiatrists display in debates over the biological or psychosocial basis of mental illnesses. Instead, pain clinics pool the knowledge and therapeutics of different specialties and allow for systematic accumulation of data that might otherwise be lost in separate specialty clinics. In addition to neurologists, psychiatrists and psychologists, there may be pharmacologists, neurosurgeons, oral surgeons, anesthesiologists, radiologists, orthopedists, neurophysiologists, physical therapists and social workers. Not every specialist is involved in every case. An oral surgeon would have little to offer in dealing with a patient with low back pain, but the contribution of each speciality is available.

In other specialty clinics and clinical departments of teaching hospitals, concepts of disease and treatment frequently become articulated in exclusionary channels, as for example in the divergence between medical and surgical treatment of ulcer. With an explicitly integrative perspective, the pain clinic has at its disposal a variety of formulations and techniques. According to Melzack (6):

> In such clinics, an interchange of ideas can occur, and the conditions are conducive to novel, imaginative approaches. Pain, in such a clinic, is not merely a symptom which each specialist perceives from his own point of view. Rather, it is the pain syndrome itself that is examined (p. 202).

The goal which binds together the diverse roles and resources of the clinic is relief of the patient's pain. The fact that a patient complaint—pain—is the common problem to which staff activities are addressed means that the attitudes and expectations of the patient receive a degree of staff attentiveness which is exceptional in the often impersonal, technological world of academic medicine and in the contemporary practice of organic medicine generally. Assessing the patient's pain may require tests and objective data. Yet the construction of an objective picture of the patient's soma remains subsidiary to the patient's own account of his distress. The significance of this can be appreciated by comparison with, for example, the typical course of medical events for a more "organic" disease such as diabetes. A patient complaint such as fainting initiates medical attention but, once the physician is on the trail of organic clues such as glucose intolerance, major emphasis shifts toward assembling the elements of an accurate, comprehensive picture of the disease. The pain clinic's preoccupation with the patient's complaint itself is probably closer to psychiatric practice in treatment of an affective problem such as anxiety or depression.

A high degree of patient-orientation on the part of the staff requires the development of clinical skills and aspects of the physician's role that are sometimes seen as having atrophied in recent years (9). Listening to the patient, interpreting the meaning of his medical problem and its place in his life, and counseling are skills of unusual importance in the pain clinic, as is the broader scope of doctor-patient communication. Unfortunately, the temper of current medical education and much medical practice runs counter to the acquisition of these competencies. Medical education conveys a great mass of biomedical information and many specific techniques from the organic side of the organic-psychic continuum, with little time or emphasis directed toward communication and relational skills. Without strong institutional support and educational preparation, pain clinicians must fashion from their own temperament, aptitudes and experience those professional skills which are essential in working with the chronic pain patient.

ROLE BALANCE BETWEEN THE PAIN PATIENT AND THE PAIN CLINIC

The interest of the pain clinic in what the patient has to say about his pain not only is a means for assessing his problem and for providing him with a sympathetic forum, important as these may be, but also provides an avenue for enlisting the patient's effort in his own treatment.

Szasz and Hollander (12) have developed a graded trichotomy of doctor-patient relationships: 1) active (doctor)/passive (patient), 2) guidance (doctor)/cooperation (patient) and 3) mutual participation. The first model has little application to pain patients, except insofar as the doctor "does something to" the patient via drugs or surgery. In the second model, the doctor tells the patient what to do and the patient obeys or cooperates. In the third model, the doctor helps the patient to help himself; his dealings with the patient are responsive to the patient's own goals and expectations for help. In their dealings with pain patients and with chronic illness patients in general, physicians probably effect a blend of the second and third Szasz-Hollander models. It is clearly desirable to enlist patient cooperation and initiative not only for the purpose of identifying the problem but also for achieving a manageable adaptation between the patient's pain disability and the larger scheme of his life.

Involving the patient in his treatment is a sociologically intricate process, which derives its rationale from the failure of earlier treatment approaches to resolve the patient's problem and from the need for new approaches.

Coming to the pain clinic is, for most pain patients, far from being their first resort to medical treatment. At one clinic in which we participated, 7 years was the average length of time during which patients had suffered significant pain. Most had previously undergone multiple surgical procedures, with little or no relief (13). The lengthy medical history of most pain clinic patients reveals their contact with specialty clinics, especially in orthopedics and neurology, and their receipt of medical treatment—medications and surgery in particular—in the first Szasz-Hollander mode. The pain clinic uses surgical and pharmacological intervention as appropriate, but its distinctive innovation consists of an approach which summons the patient's involvement and personal resources for coping with pain. Under earlier regimes, by definition not lastingly successful, the patient typically turned his problem over to a physician who assumed major responsibility. Thus, the chronic patient who presents himself at a pain clinic as a rule quickly notices a contrast, by comparison with earlier experience, in what is expected of him.

We stated above that the sick-role contains within it the element of seeking professional care. A person does not fully enter into the sick-role so long as he is dealing with his illness only in his own terms. What happens, then, if a sick person goes to a physician—as in a pain clinic—who in turn hands back to him an important part of the responsibility for dealing with his problem?

It is at this point that the complexity of the role balance between patient and physician in the treatment process becomes apparent. If the pain professional restores to a help-seeking patient the responsibility for coping with his problem, then, from a simplistic standpoint, everything would seem much as it was before the patient came. The professional's attitude could be construed as: "There is nothing—unfortunately—that I can do for you. Therefore I leave you to your own devices. Good luck!" In the medical history of many pain patients, something similar to this may have happened during earlier interventions with drugs or surgery: the physician has done something rather than nothing, but once he exhausted his pharmaceutical or surgical remedies he discharged the patient still in distress.

A more accurate statement of what happens at the pain clinic is that, in arousing patient participation and initiative in treatment, the clinic still retains responsibility in terms of clinical oversight, but it redefines the ongoing responsibility which the patient is asked to accept. The sick-role formulation, by which the sick person takes his problem to a professional for help, retains its cogency, although to it must be annexed the provision that the ensuing state of affairs includes a sharing of responsibility by the sick person and the professional rather than unilateral professional assumption of responsibility. This eventuality is distinctly recognized by Parsons (8) in an expanded analysis of the sick-role, in which he noted that the patient in the context of health care agencies is not merely the passive object of treatment. Notwithstanding the fact that acutely ill individuals in treatment might find their own activities minimized . . .

. . . the less acute the immediate situation, the more likely it is that (the patient's) participation will be substantial. It may concentrate on a role complementary to that of the health care agent in furthering the goal of either recovery or minimization of the curtailment of the capacities of the healthy person (p. 28).

The kinds of participation which may be expected of a pain clinic patient are varied: acquiring control over autonomic functions through biofeedback training, physical exercise, self-hypnosis and individual or group psychotherapy. The role of staff reflects their own expectations of the patient. Instead of the traditional hierarchical imbalance between staff and patient, the staff role allows and requires greater scope for counseling, encouraging and challenging the patient.

Work with chronic pain patients fosters a gradual yet radical reshaping of the traditional concept of medical responsibility which is the motivational root for much physician behavior (10). Instead of responsibility linked to control over technological, intellectual, and organizational resources, the pain clinician practices a less obsessive and dominance-oriented order of responsibility toward the patient. In this respect as in many others, the practice of "pain medicine" goes against the grain of much in contemporary medicine.

PATIENT SELF-CONCEPT

Applied to chronic patients, the parsonian sick-role concept is expanded, although not fundamentally violated, in its account of what is involved when the patient seeks professional help. There is another component of the sick-role which requires special scrutiny in relation to chronic pain patients, namely, the premise that the patient's problem—that is, his pain— is "not his fault." As we have noted, the sick person is entitled to sympathy and respect. He is protected from social condemnation and loss of dignity. Reflexively, his self-concept, which tends to mirror the evaluation of him by others, is shielded from guilt, shame and other uncomfortable feelings.

Tremendous social leverage is attached to full-fledged occupancy of the sick-role. The sick person, as well as his protectors and advocates, will tend to support his sick-role status against threats and demeaning claims.

Some kinds of illness, even with unquestionable medical etiology, are stigmatized and do not confer full sick-role benefits. Venereal disease is a leading example. Negative social attitudes may hold that the VD patient deserves his troubles; another telling indication of stigma is the limited amount of biomedical effort directed toward the development of gonorrhea vaccines.

Similar issues arise in regard to mental illness in general and schizophrenia in particular. Along with its clinical efforts on behalf of individual patients, the psychiatric profession as a whole has developed historically within medicine on the premise that mental illness is a sickness which entitles its bearers to sick-role occupancy and to treatment, which is frequently non-specific. Whatever their scientific validity, theories of schizophrenia (and other major mental illnesses) which trace it to a biochemical deficiency or genetic defect play a critical social function by legitimizing the illness—by stating, implicitly, that it is not the patient's fault nor anyone else's. Parents of schizophrenic children may find it relatively more acceptable to think that their child's difficulty is due to genetic factors rather than emotionally possessive or impulsive child-rearing practices. In other words, concepts of the origin and course of an illness can have important social consequences for the sick person. Even the treatment used for an illness may carry with it implications as to the origin and nature of the illness, again with social consequences bearing upon the legitimacy and associated benefits of sick-role occupancy and the social reputation of the sick person.

Similarly, there are fundamental questions about the nature of pain which, in addition to their important place in the scheme of biological investigation, have major social consequences for the pain sufferer—for how others regard him and for how he regards himself. By extension these questions have important implications for the organization and rationale of clinical efforts to deal with pain, as in pain clinics.

Many pain clinic patients have had great difficulty in sustaining a sick-role identity. In one pain clinic in which we participated, much of the opening session was given over to validating the pain role. "We *know* you hurt," the director insisted. "We know it isn't just in your head." This seemed of immense value to the patients, some of whom appeared to have expended a fair amount of energy in the past defending their right to a sick-role in the face of physicians' refusal to legitimate it. The chronic pain patient, perhaps more often than other chronically ill or disabled patients, often has need for official validation not only for the benefit of his social situation but also in case of litigation following automobile accidents or occupational injury and disability payments of various types based on inability to work. This can conceivably complicate the prognosis, by offering a valuable secondary gain.

As the director of one of the new pain clinics, Sternbach (11), has stated, "Should the magic bullet appear which would abolish all pain, a very significant proportion of chronic pain patients would continue to complain of pain and indeed 'have' it by all objective criteria. This is because they have so altered their lives that they need the pain and cannot live without it" (p. 123).

Consequently, in the Sternbach clinic, patients are asked to go over their typical day in detail and to note what they would lose if they did not have their pain—in work, domestic life, disability compensation, sympathetic attention, exemption from sexual expectation and release from care for others. What would be changed in the patient's life if he or she could get rid of the pain? For many patients, pain provides abundant benefits. Although highly unpleasant, pain can have a self-sustaining continuity for the patient; it is familiar, and it is authentically his own. In the ramifications of interpersonal relationships, particularly those in the family, significant others may become stably attuned to the chronic painful state of a sick relative or friend. It is familiar to them also, and in their interactions they may not project the adaptive, recovery-oriented version of the sick-role but rather may project a deviant, dependency-maximizing version of it.

SOCIOLOGICAL IMPLICATIONS OF PAIN THEORY

While it is unwise to overinterpret or descry a monolithic intellectual attitude among the medical pioneers who have established pain clinics and are shaping multidisciplinary perspectives on pain, it appears that there is a general shared emphasis upon the likelihood that patients can modify their experience of pain. Under this concept, modification is to be accomplished through learning, training and practice in techniques of focusing, interrupting and reflecting the awareness of pain. It is not to be accomplished through a sheer act of will or determination, which would tend to delegitimize the patient's sick-role status. Suppressive tactics may, however, be employed; in her description of a pain clinic, Wrobel (13) reports that patients are asked not to mention their pain during group sessions (although they may do so in private sessions with counselors).

Most pain investigators and therapists accept the distinction between pain sensation and pain experience—that the patient's suffering is not the direct registration of a painful sensation but rather is formed by anticipations, perceptions and emotional reactions in relation to a noxious sensation. Particular attention is paid to past learning as constituting a matrix within which the patient presently responds to pain. Sometimes the relevant learning is conceived to occur early in the individual's life—so that the adult's response to internal pain stimuli is an elaboration or repetition of reactions to childhood traumas. Alternatively, the relevant learning is viewed as contemporaneous with the onset of the illness or insult which started the pain—as, for example, when an arthritis patient feels severe pain in anticipation of an attack. Whether the learning that contributes to the pain experience is biographically early or late, the significant implication for professional practice with pain patients is that what is learned can be unlearned or overlaid with new learning that obsolesces previous patterns.

Zborowski's (14, 15) classic anthropological study of ethnically differentiated pain tolerance among hospitalized veterans fits within the general intellectual framework of human response to pain as a form of learned behavior. His finding—that there are characteristic differences between

Old-America, Irish, Italian and Jewish patients in their attitude toward and response to pain—argues strongly that individuals learn pain response in culturally patterned ways.

In the first part of *People in Pain*, Zborowski (15) develops the idea that pain is a biological universal which, like hunger and sex, becomes the basis for varying patterns of cultural behavior. Pain behavior, like eating behavior, is culturally shaped from a biological base. In building his case for cultural variation, Zborowski draws upon the earlier contributions of medical pain investigators such as Beecher, Wolff, Bonica, Cannon and Engel. It is interesting to note, however, that the current clinically oriented pain literature pays little attention to cultural variation. This may be in part because, as Zborowski suggests, "Members of the medical profession are reluctant to differentiate patients according to religion, race, or nationality" (p. 4). Ethnicity or other social group differences are seen as medically irrelevant, although Zborowski found that physicians did have strong impressions, corresponding closely to the findings of his own subsequent research, about how patients of different ethnic groups responded to pain.

In addition to the individualizing stance which clinical medicine adopts toward each patient, we suggest an additional reason for lack of interest in cultural variation. Although cultural variation certainly stems from transmitted and learned patterns, there is nothing that the individual patient, nor the pain clinic, can do about the patient's ethnicity or any other group membership category—regardless of how relevant such categories may be in understanding the patient's response to pain. The cultural perspective seems to offer no scope for clinical intervention.

Psychological approaches based upon the biographical particulars of a patient's learning about pain in his childhood and later life are in greater favor, although it is not clear that the patient is in a better position to do anything about such learning than he is about his ethnicity. Nevertheless, individualistic biographical approaches probably feed the aura of hope for clinical improvement more effectively than would a cultural approach.

The concept that an individual has "learned his way" into life difficulties provides a strong motivational platform for efforts on the part of both the individual himself and his professional helpers to extricate him from his difficulties. Quite aside from the scientific merit of concepts of learned pain behavior, such concepts comport with therapeutic optimism. Further, learned behavior is viewed as not immediately voluntary and yet as modifiable—hence susceptible to clinically guided amelioration. The learning perspective thus protects the right of the pain patient to be viewed as the victim of his condition, occupying the sick-role without stigma or rejection.

Pain Treatment and Contemporary Trends in Medicine

We have suggested above that the pain clinic is a novel organization of medical services, which combines diverse clinical specialties, new theoretical concepts of pain and nontraditional models of the doctor-patient relationship. The multidisciplinary work of pain clinics is an attempt to combine accepted interventions, as necessary, from neurosurgery and pharmacology with clinical expertise in individualized, patient-oriented education and counseling.

Professional work with chronic pain patients falls well within the scope of therapy-oriented health professional roles yet represents a particular expression of the general therapeutic role. Absolute cure of the patient's pain problem is always the most desirable result but, where this is out of reach, relief is still a realistic objective in many cases. There is a lack of concepts and accepted vocabulary for identifying precisely the kinds of staff orientation and skills which are mobilized and articulated in the process of helping chronic pain patients, although they clearly lie within the area of rehabilitation and education. Medical professionals who work in the area of pain do so without the firm identity supports which come from carrying out specialized, technical medical tasks learned in the prevailing structure of medical education.

Innovation in medicine frequently arouses scepticism and derision in critics. When "psychological" means are used to deal with a "physical" problem such as pain, charges of quackery and charlatanism are quick in coming. Melzack (6) was well aware of this when he noted that the historical emphasis on sensory mechanisms and the relative neglect of motivational and cognitive variables in pain had made effective therapies such as tranquillizers, suggestions, placebos and hypnosis seem suspect or even "fraudulent, almost a sideshow in the mainstream of pain treatment."

In attempting to provide relief for the chronic pain patient, pain clinics and personnel can be seen as part of a larger trend—strong, though uneven and certainly not unified in overall impact—to supplement medical technology with interpersonal influence and communication within institutional settings that adhere to the clinical model of patient and doctor (assisted, of course, by other health professionals). Broadly analogous developments are occurring as health professionals, dealing with major chronic diseases such as diabetes and hypertension, recognize the great need to supplement medical intervention with instruction and counseling for patients in nutrition, physical activity and other aspects of daily living. Like patients with chronic diseases, the chronic pain sufferer must also achieve improvement not through cure but through building a life which respects limitations imposed by physicians without becoming exhaustively defined by them. In time, new roles for patient and professional will evolve, as will new sociomedical institutions and processes created for these purposes.

Acknowledgment

The authors wish to express their appreciation to Maureen Searle for her critical reading of successive drafts and for her helpful editorial suggestions.

REFERENCES

1. BEECHER, H. K. *Measurement of Subjective Responses.* Oxford University Press, New York, 1959.
2. FAGERHAUGH, S., AND STRAUSS, A. *Politics of Pain Management: Staff-Patient Interaction.* Addison-Wesley Publishing Company, Menlo Park, CA, 1977.
3. FREIDSON, E. The sociology of medicine: A trend report and bibliography. *Curr. Sociol., 10/11:* 125, 1961–1962.
4. FOX, R. C. The medicalization and demedicalization of American society. *Daedalus, 106:* 9–22, 1977.
5. GALLAGHER, E. B. Lines of extension and reconstruction in the parsonian sociology of illness. *Soc. Sci. Med., 10:* 207–218, 1976.
6. MELZACK, R. *The Puzzle of Pain.* Basic Books, New York, 1973.
7. PARSONS, T. *The Social System.* Free Press, Glencoe, IL, 1951.
8. PARSONS, T. *Action Theory and the Human Condition.* Macmillan-Free Press, New York, 1978.
9. REISER, S. J. *Medicine and the Reign of Technology.* Cambridge University Press, Cambridge, 1978.
10. SEARLE, M. Medical Responsibility: Insights into Medical Behavior. Unpublished paper, Yale University Department of Sociology, 1980.
11. STERNBACH, R. *Pain Patients: Traits and Treatment.* Academic Press, New York, 1974.
12. SZASZ, T., AND HOLLANDER, M. A contribution to the philosophy of medicine: The basic models of the doctor-patient relationship. *A. M. A. Arch. Intern. Med., 97:* 585–592, 1956.
13. WROBEL, S. Quiet battle. *The Courier Journal Magazine.* Louisville, KT, June 11, 1978.
14. ZBOROWSKI, M. Cultural components in response to pain. *J. Soc. Iss. 8:* 16–30, 1952.
15. ZBOROWSKI, M. *People in Pain.* Jossey-Bass, San Francisco, 1969.

5

Chronic Pain and the Occupational Role

ELDON TUNKS, M.D.
RANJAN ROY, Adv. Dip. S.W.

There is an often told story of a question being posed to Sigmund Freud, asking him what the essential criteria of normality were, and his response was simply "love and work." In this succinct answer, he said much; to have health, both the interpersonal relationships and the occupational role must be satisfactory and in balance. The purpose of this chapter is to look at the occupational role and the changes and stresses imposed on it by chronic pain and illness. No one would argue that the occupational role has a powerful integrating effect on human behavior, that an individual dispossessed of this role is apt to be in great difficulty, and that permitting someone to return to this role may be the most important single step in rehabilitation.

Human roles are those behavioral programs which are carried out by individuals according to societal expectations and rules; they are stable over time, allow for predictability and are compatible with the rules governing others in the environment, and the roles are complementary to roles of others within that ecological system. Roles serve the purpose of maintaining social order by reducing dissonance or distress, allowing for adaptation, and providing a basis for satisfaction. Therefore, a loss or a major change of role may have the effect of causing the individual to be identified as deviant or sick, may interfere with his adaptation, may produce distress or dissatisfaction, and may change other roles that that individual simultaneously carries. Concomitantly, when a loss or change of role occurs in one individual in the system, there will be a parallel shift in role expectations affecting individuals contiguous to the index member. The system of individuals in the ecology may become destabilized, the individuals may experience dissonance and dissatisfaction, and there may be impairment of group functioning and adaptation, with consequent further effect on the index member. These interdependent role changes are necessitated by the complementarity that exists in an ecological system and by virtue of the rules which govern not only the index individuals but also the others in the environment. Change leads to shifts which produce a new complementarity; this change occurs in an orderly fashion according to the rules which existed there beforehand. There is always an interplay such that the system as a whole—the index individual in the context with the ecology—must be considered.

Role Types

As suggested above, each individual has a variety of roles; these must be compatible with each other, and there is an interaction between the roles maintained by any one individual, and an interaction between the roles of a particular individual and those of others in the ecology. Roles might be arbitrarily categorized in terms of familial, occupational, societal, and personal roles (6). Obviously, each of these four categories might be further broken down into a number of subcategories.

For example, the family roles maintained by an individual may include being father to one's children, husband to a wife, child to parents, and a member of an extended family to a nephew; in a short space of time, appropriate role behavior demonstrated by an individual in a family system may show all of these different facets. An important part of family role function is that of "the provider" and this provides an important linkage to another set of roles categorized as the occupational roles. The latter in turn have a number of subcategories such as being at the service of the employer, a co-worker with one's peers, a committee member charged with certain functions, a shop steward, etc. Societal roles likewise are multiple and define a wide range of behaviors that are expected from an individual as he moves within the ecological system. The appropriate role behavior of a defendant in a court fits the rules and expectations laid down by society and is complementary with roles of court personnel, judges and lawyers. The same individual who appears in court may the following day be a patient with all that implies as he waits in the doctor's office, a client to be pleased in a shop, and one of a group to be bargained with in a citizen's committee. (Below, we will be giving particular attention to the illness role and its relationship to other societal, occupational, family and personal role systems.) The fourth category of roles is that of "personal role behavior." (This might alternatively be called internalized expectations and values.) This sort of behavior perhaps is less obvious than, for example, occupational or family roles but is of equal importance, and it defines that set of behaviors by which an individual actualizes personal expectations according to sets of personal rules that have been acquired during growth and development. The identity assumed is in relationship to the range of interpersonal experiences that have shaped growth and development, in relationship to objects of the ego, and decisions that have been made along the way. As the individual strives toward actualizing that set of expectations, he is fulfilling his need for mastery, his need to earn leisure, his need to be in control of contingencies affecting his life, and his need to be able to ward off threat or sources of anxiety. Personal role, therefore, is very much tied up with one's concept of oneself, and playing it out successfully determines the achievement of satisfaction, or lack of it.

Roles in Relationship to Illness

Although there is a great deal of description and research regarding issues of acute and chronic pain, pain mechanisms and treatment, there is a relative poverty of data concerning illness roles, particularly with respect to chronic pain. For example, in several studies concerned with the outcome of treatment, the outcome was measured in terms of analgesic intake, levels of activity, and reported changes in pain severity, etc., all obviously relevant to functioning but giving only a preliminary view of the psychosocial situation and how it changed (4, 10, 14). A number of assumptions are made, perhaps without adequate foundation. For example, Shealy (11) reported that divorce was high amongst patients with chronic pain, but no evidence was offered to satisfactorily show that pain was the only significant factor contributing to the marital breakdown nor did there appear to have been an exploration of the state of the marriage before the onset of the pain problem. Another sort of assumption is that if pain becomes intractable, all role function may be discarded and the patient may become "firmly entrenched in the sick role." That this is not necessarily so has been demonstrated by Pilowsky and Spence (8) in a study in which a group of older women with intractable pain were found to have continued a number of daily social commitments despite their pain. These individuals were, in general, similar to other pain patients on the Illness Behavior Questionnaire (IBQ) except that they were somewhat less irritable. A paper by Seres and Newman (10) also cast doubt on the equation of chronicity and abandonment of all appropriate roles. The psychosocial consequence of treatment has also been a neglected subject. While on the one hand it is a common observation that individuals will do well in a treatment program if they have been socially well adjusted (12), it is not clear whether as a rule individuals completely resume their roles and functioning after apparently adequate treatment and reasonable pain relief.

A lot of difficulty in evaluating the psychosocial response to illness and treatment comes from an inordinate concentration on the capacity for work as an essential criterion of outcome. Certainly that criterion is important because of social cost and because of special interest by insurance plans and Workmen's Compensation Boards and costs to industry for example, but to interpret the abrogation of the breadwinner role as implying a global loss of roles and functions may be a hasty generalization (5, 9, 15). Sternbach (12) regarded the factor of returning to work as a measure of treatment outcome too stringent an application of the work ethic. To put the question around the other way, the maintenance of the occupational role despite the presence of chronic illness or pain might be considered to be a criterion predicting a good prognosis in treatment. It is a common observation that patients who have continued to work but who are showing the disrupting effects of pain in their personal and family lives are apt to do better in a treatment program than other individuals who have also stopped working.

What one gathers from all of the above is that despite the many unanswered questions, one can safely say that chronic pain in particular has a disrupting effect to various degrees on ability to maintain adequate working behavior, position in society and family, and ideal personal function. In all of this the occupational role plays a very important part, being destabilized by the stress of pain and illness but at the same time, if maintained, providing a protective influence and interacting with other functions. Hasty generalizations should not be made nor should loss of function be considered absolute in all areas.

More specific attention should at this time be focused on the issue of chronicity and the complexities that it introduces. On the one hand, in the case of acute illness there is the common assumption that pathology of a definable sort exists in proportion to the complaint and in proportion to the loss of function, and that a complaint will lead to a therapeutic intervention which relieves the disorder so that the person can resume functioning once the pathology is eradicated. But when irreversible pathological damage, residual disabilities, or complaints in the absence of easily definable pathology are encountered, differences are encountered between the "acute sick-role" and the "chronic sick-role" (1, 5). In the latter case, the patient may never be able to complete the move out of the sick-role—resumption of some roles would be impossible or even inadvisable. This immediately puts this individual at odds with societal and individual expectations. In fact, the needs of the health team, family, or the patient himself may even cause the individual to accept an "obligation to remain sick" to legitimize the inability to return to the pre-illness condition. Some degree of compensation may be developed by the patient toward his chronic disorder as he accepts his condition and learns to manage his own treatment and rehabilitation within the limits of what his physician can delegate to him. He may acquire skills in self-medication and diet, in using prostheses, in performing tests of his bodily functions, in caring for his therapeutic equipment and so on. While the patient is no longer able to meet his usual premorbid obligations, he now has a new set of obligations; society at large (which includes his own family) may have different expectations, with a result that there may be tension and hostility.

A 35-year-old farmer suffered multiple fractures and injuries when struck by a carelessly driven truck. Afterward he continued to suffer from chronic back pain and incapacity to resume his normal farm work, and he was in receipt of payments from

the insurer of the motor vehicle. After more than a year, when his physical c
was no longer improving and before the litigation was settled, the man took
advice of consulting physicians who were telling him that he might have to "learn to
live with it." Although not productive as he was before, he began to apply himself to
various tasks about the farm and to increase the amount of active time by spending
time out of doors throughout the day. He was dismayed to receive notice that
officials of the insuring company had begun to take clandestine photographs of him
as he was on his property, using this as evidence of his recovery.

On the other hand an individual may not undergo new learning and
compensation and may go on behaving in a way which is more characteristic
of an acute illness response—seeking out diagnoses and cures—and being
shuttled about as an incurable. (This question is dealt with in more detail
in Chapter 4 by Gallagher and Wrobel.)

The Chronic Pain Patient Versus the Occupational Role

Implicit in the occupational role is that the individual must demonstrate
motivation to render the hired service, must share responsibilities with
other employees, and must receive fair recompense, promotion and recognition, and security of tenure. A problem such as chronic pain may be
incompatible with continuation of this occupational role, with the consequence that occupational dysfunction or loss results in loss of pay, of
promotion, of respect, and of security. (Health professionals such as those
reading this chapter might forget that the majority of occupations performed
by society members at large are not particularly fulfilling and enjoyable on
a day-to-day basis and may even be quite unpleasant. The social status that
goes along with the job and factors such as shift work may make the job
and the activity associated with it unsatisfying and frustrating so that pain
may become the obvious, but not necessarily the single, cause of inability to
return to the work place.) The employer, whose place is complementary to
that of the employee, may now regard the disabled individual as a poor risk
and as unmotivated. The existence of "sick leave plans" has little in the way
of a mitigating effect on such a process of reevaluation of the employee since
demonstration of illness is not a part of expected employee behavior. Sick-
leave plans or Workmen's Compensation agreements may in fact have an
aggravating effect by imposing an "obligation to remain sick." For example
a patient may be persuaded to enter a rehabilitation program involving,
among other things, work placement and occupational therapy for problems
of chronic pain and disability. Medical reports may be sent according to
regulation to the insuring board or insurance company. The patient may
then suddenly find that his benefits have been cut on the grounds that if he
can participate so many hours per week in a rehabilitation program then he
must no longer be totally disabled. The final result of this may be panic and
deterioration in the level of functioning and failure of the rehabilitation

program. It is important to note that even when disincentives for recovery are avoided, chronic pain patients have often built up a great deal of suspicion.

Workmen's Compensation Boards (W.C.B.), sick-leave insurance, and other benefits from collective bargaining agreements are all in place with the purpose of improving the status of the workman and relationships with which he must deal, but in the presence of a problem of chronic pain the same agreements can serve to set the stage for adversary relationships. We might mention at this point that we have had the occasion to see several injured workmen who had been shop stewards prior to their injuries; the degree of adversary relationship between these individuals and their employers and other agencies was perceptibly aggravated in these cases.

Workmen's Compensation Boards are also an integral part of the occupational ecology: W.C.B. intervention makes the disabled employee a financial liability to the company. At the same time, the injured workman is a statistic to the W.C.B. which must minimize or eliminate individuals on its caseload if it is to maintain its credibility. This is not to slander Workmen's Compensation Boards but rather to point out the dilemma of mixed loyalty into which they are forced. Meanwhile, the W.C.B. is frequently a target for the injured workman's anger when he perceives the benefits received as being a pittance instead of resembling a just compensation and, therefore, there is another interface for an adversary relationship.

If an employee has developed a record of recurrent or long-term health problems, the employer may prefer to keep him out of the shop regardless of any medical information that may be supplied to the Personnel Office. Further, the medical department of the company may in many cases simply function as the "hatchet man" for the Personnel Office. (Fortunately, this state of affairs is not always so, but in many small companies it is still distressingly true.) The employer may reduce potential liability for sick leave and W.C.B. assessments by creating a condition for return to work which is prohibitive to the employee; offering inappropriate work to the injured workman even though more appropriate jobs may be available, thereby putting the workman in the position of either resigning or of being fired for not being able to perform.

A specific example encountered by the authors was that of an individual who had been regarded with suspicion by his company after he was injured on the job and had remained off work on W.C.B. benefits for several months. The company offered this man a different job in the lowest level of management, which would have taken him out of the bargaining unit and out of the protection of the Union. This injured employee had heard it rumored from workmates that the company would use any excuse to fire him, and he found himself on the horns of the dilemma; if he accepted the job, he ran the risk of being fired shortly afterward, but if he did not accept the job he ran the risk of appearing unmotivated. Rather than take the risk, he eventually found a management position in a completely different company where he functioned well.

Another important part of the occupation ecology is the Union to which the worker belongs. Intervention by the Union on behalf of the injured employee may force the hand of the employer, but at the cost of creating an adversary relationship which is intimidating to the employee. Faced with this and with the further discouragement of a long wait, the employee may afterward find himself returned to a hostile setting incompatible with receiving the recognition, promotion, and security that he would otherwise expect. It should furthermore be mentioned that hostility toward an injured employee is not confined to the employer but may also come from other employees sharing that part of the shop and may come from the foreman who is under obligation to management to be productive.

Relationship to Family Roles

When the occupational role fails, the provider role also fails, resulting in a shift of other familial roles as the adjustment and redistribution of the provider function take place. The fact that the injured individual may be in receipt of benefits (which rarely provide much better than subsistence living) may pit the family against "the system" and may additionally give rise to intrafamilial discontent. That discontent may not be clearly or directly expressed, however, because the set of rules that govern response to an ill person evoke the opposite behaviors of sympathy and rescue.

Normally, in a family the provider maintains his full spousal and parental role partly by virtue of the security that the occupational role brings. When the occupational role is dysfunctional or lost, there is a shift of expectations. For example, the spouse of the injured partner may now regard the disabled member as a dependent in the same way as an aged parent or child would be regarded; such change in perception would produce mutual role dissatisfaction and could even lead to family dissolution. Parent-child relationships are also affected frequently, with the disabled member being sidelined from family function. Such an effect is not necessarily implicit in the disability but rather is symbolic of the now devitalized parental role.

A 40-year-old immigrant workman was injured and developed chronic neck pain. The wife obtained a job because W.C.B. benefits were insufficient to cover the cost of raising four school-age children, paying a mortgage and maintaining a decent standard of living. The husband, however, did not see it as being part of his role to increase his child-care and household-based function, so that the wife now found herself with both the breadwinner role and an expanded role as parent. After a further period of time, the wife also began to develop medical complaints which she attributed to her husband's prolonged disability, and she left her job. When they presented in the Pain Clinic, his chief complaint was that his chronic neck pain and headache were making his life insufferable and that he was "nervous" because he was no longer a man. Her complaint was that she had become ill and "nervous" because she could not cope with four small children and a grown-up one plus a job all at the same time.

Relationship to Personal Roles

As discussed above, this is the field of expectations and self-perceptions that arise during growth and development, and on this is predicated the sense of mastery. It involves expectations of being able to earn one's leisure, to control contingencies affecting one's life, and to ward off threat. The loss of the occupational role threatens all of this; the new position is dissonant and dissatisfying and, faced with this, the individual may well retreat to role behaviors held earlier during growth and development. The regressed role may be characterized by a show of dependency (clinging to other family members and agencies for security), a needy and clamoring posture (for example, exaggerated pain complaint), and a defeated and passive position which is complementary to the expectation that others in the ecology will take an active rescuer position (12). With this personal role shift and all of its attendant dissatisfaction, there is a concomitant shift in family and environmental role behavior, with further reinforcing impact upon the index individual. The injured person is apt to regard the events leading to the role change as catastrophic and the process as irreversible. This might be illustrated in findings by Woodforde and Merskey (18) who noted that injured individuals demonstrated more signs of neuroticism, anxiety, and depression than did a psychiatric group who were experiencing pain without apparent physical cause. The former group, furthermore, saw themselves as having been prior to their injuries well-adjusted, stable, successful, and well-controlled; they appeared to overvalue their perceptions of their previous character as stable and ideal in a response to the awareness that they had probably become more psychologically vulnerable and distressed.

In the foregoing paragraph, consideration was given to the effect of chronic illness and loss of work upon the individual. One must also, however, consider effect of growth and development and characterological variables in the eventual acquisition of pain and disability. In his classic paper entitled "Psychogenic Pain and the Pain Prone Patient," Engel (3) cites a number of examples with discussion of how the problem of pain becomes the crystallization of conflictual problems, and problems in object relations. Pain becomes an interpersonal communication and, as Szasz (15, 16) pointed out, that communication may in a sense be more significant than the biological event to which the pain is attributed by the patient. It should also be remembered that chronic pain sufferers may be more likely to have family members who selectively respond to illness communications, thereby perpetuating a system in which the ill posture will be maintained (2, 17).

It should be noted again that with the advent of chronic illness or chronic pain one does not necessarily see the abandonment of roles. What one sees involves in various individuals different degrees of loss of certain role functions and alterations of others.

Case Study

A 35-year-old unmarried man was referred to the Pain Clinic for complaints of chronic sciatica and chronic depression. As a young adult he had immigrated with his parents and siblings to Canada and had obtained work. A few years later he was injured and was unable to carry on as a laborer. A rehabilitation program 10 years previously had arranged for him to go to a light laboring job, where he had continued to the present with some sick time. Since his injury he had ceased all socializing and had no longer associated with women. He lived in the Y.M.C.A. and once every 2 weeks he would go to another town to see his parents. Virtually all of his free time was spent in solitude; on occasion, he would ring up his physician. His explanation of why he had continued to live such an isolated existence was that with his chronic sciatica he could never offer stability and security to a family and he saw himself as being an undesirable mate for any marriage. He continued to cling to the thought that should his pain be cured some day he might then return to a normal existence. He steadfastly refused to visit old friends because, he said, they had now married, and he did not wish to impose himself. Inquiry by the examiner of the employer revealed that sick time currently being taken was beyond the tolerable limit and that the employer had considered terminating this employee if sick time increased, even for reasons of medical treatment.

The examiner was of the opinion that this man had been rather passive even premorbidly, and that now after his injury he had withdrawn from all but the occupational setting, some minimal family contact and occasional visits to a physician. Physician contacts were at this time offering him one of his only avenues for affective communication, albeit expressed in terms of physical distress and depression. On a direct challenge the patient admitted that, even should the illness no longer be present, it would be unlikely he should make any fundamental changes, and he recognized that there must be some problem in the way he viewed himself in relation to others.

In the above example the event of injury precipitated in this individual a set of changes that were partly dependent on his character structure and cultural milieu but that, the way he recalled it, were importantly determined by his loss of ability to carry out his original job. He recalled his period of unemployment and disability with great unhappiness and saw his current position as tenuous. At least the way he saw it, lacking job security on account of his sciatica, he was unwilling to engage himself in anything more than a minimal interpersonal existence. These interdependent role changes had involved the role of patient (jeopardizing the role of worker), had affected personal role functioning and had markedly limited his familial and social role functioning.

Relationship to Societal Roles—The Patient Role

In the event of illness, the role of patient may be assumed. This essentially represents a new role for most individuals, but it is not foreign or unknown to the ecology nor vicariously to the index individual, and there are preexistent rules governing the events that follow. The illness brings that individual into contact with healing or rehabilitation professions, and for the sake of the discussion we shall focus on the physician as representative of the helper professions. The patient presents with his complaint and expresses the wish to be cured. During the acute stages of illness, this is appropriate role behavior and usually leads to recovery after prescribed treatment and convalescence. This situation is compatible with the expectation that the patient should be supplicant to the healer. Also defined in this situation is that the focus should be on the pathophysiology as the source of distress, and so the process of diagnosis and cure is carried out. In the case of chronic but definable pathophysiology, the emphasis may have to change to amelioration of the illness process, modification of distress, and a learning experience in which the patient accepts responsibility as much as possible for his own care and for some degree of adjustment to life responsibilities. More complicated is the situation in which an individual continues to have chronic pain after the original injury is long passed, with relatively little definable pathophysiology to support the complaint. In such a situation the supplicant is simultaneously experiencing dissatisfaction in a dissonant system of overlapping ecologies. The process of his adaptation may be dependent on more than resolution of the pathophysiological process and may require a more satisfactory resolution of the multiple role changes or restoration of functioning to a less dissonant pattern. Fortuitously, in many cases, medical intervention is followed by sufficient alleviation of symptoms and signs, and in most cases the occupational role and other functioning are reestablished. Such good outcome is often as much good fortune as it is good management, because rarely in the consulting room is the scope of the whole disability problem considered. Too often, therefore, when treatment fails the unfortunate results depend not so much on whether the medical practice was carried on correctly but more on the multiple dissatisfactions into which the individual has been precipitated.

When the "medical failure" occurs, there is also a new dissonance—the physician's expectation is to be successful just as the patient's expectation is to be cured. When such happy outcome does not occur, there is mutual dissatisfaction, and the physician may question the patient's motivation or even his sanity. The epithets with which this is done may include such things as "compensation neurosis," which translates to "you are bilking the system," or "hysteria," which translates to "you are a coward and weakling," or "hysteromalingering," which means "you are a liar," or politely "psychogenic pain," which may mean "you are imagining it or even crazy" (9). It is notable at this point that the supplicant is still not considered in other than the patient role and he is still being given labels and evaluations confirming him in the patient role but is now regarded as displaying unacceptable patient behavior, with complaints in excess of obvious findings, and is being recategorized as a less desirable patient. Both doctor and patient may retrench; the physician may make an effort to send the patient back to work and, therefore, may be regarded with suspicion by the patient, but the patient may passively go through the motions of returning and then visit the physician's office shortly afterward complaining of aggravation, necessitating reevaluation, rediagnosis, and attempted cure. The physician may feel angry and "used" in being asked to validate the patient's disability by answering letters or filling out W.C.B. forms or by having to certify when his patient will or will no longer be disabled. The physician role is at the same time under pressure from societal norms and pressure from other agencies to take action to resolve the illness problem and remove the patient from the illness role. Such expectation often leads to lateral moves of the patient through a consultative referral system, further perpetuating the ill role.

Case Discussion

To attempt illustration of foregoing considerations, the following case is described in some detail.

This 52-year-old man had worked for 20 years in a large manufacturing firm as a laborer and had built up a good deal of experience and seniority before he experienced a back injury. For a while he was off work and in receipt of W.C.B. payments and then returned to a light job at a lower classification selected for him by the Company. Shortly afterwards, he was reinjured as a result of horseplay by workmates and was off work on a new W.C.B. claim, this time for a longer period of time. Apparently, the patient expressed some bitterness to the Company that he had been put on the job where he was reinjured. The Company then suggested to him another position within the plant; one that involved a fair amount of stooping and lifting. According to the Company, this job was perfectly compatible with medical reports that had been received by the medical office.

The injured workman had begun to see himself as being victimized by reason of having been injured, and the adversary feeling was building but probably was not yet irreversible. The third job now offered to this patient probably was in fact inappropriate and it was reasonable to believe that there had come about some breakdown in understanding between the medical evaluations which had been sent in only by letter and their interpretation at the Company side.

When the patient was returned to a heavy job, conflict broke out within 2 days regarding the appropriateness of the new position, with the patient complaining to the Union about the Company and Workmen's Compensation Board, and the Workmen's Compensation Board complaining to the Company, with the result that the patient had a "chip on his shoulder" about Workmen's Compensation Board and was mistrustful of the Company; following this, there was no employment for 2 years.

By now there was significant embarrassment of family functioning and marital stress, and this man was showing depression and frustration with unfruitful medical interventions. Through the referral system he finally arrived at the Pain Clinic and was referred to the Inpatient Pain Behavior Modification Unit where a 6-week contract was established "to increase the level of occupational activity regardless of pain level" by use of work stations in hospital workshops, exercise program with increasing expectations for activity output, general relaxation training, and group education (therapy). Analgesics were modified and reduced.

By the sixth week he had dropped his adversary posture toward W.C.B. and Company and before discharge in informal meetings had arrived at a verbal agreement between a lesser officer in the Personnel Department of his company and Workmen's Compensation Board to soon return to his old department to one of several available light jobs. He followed the required procedure of contacting the medical department and having the appropriate forms submitted to the Personnel Department. When time began to drag on with no word being received, inquiry was made to the Company, and the response indicated that management and foremen were trading subtle messages that they had the right to refuse an employee who may be a poor risk.

Once an individual has become stigmatized as a "chronic" and "unable to work," the economics and politics of the working place environment may militate against his being able to change that posture. It is at a point such as this that many patients revert to their previous adversary and angry stance and forego any further chance of being returned to the able role.

Pressure brought to bear by the Union and W.C.B. together led to the Personnel Office offering a few rather heavy and inappropriate jobs at low pay scales outside the section in which the workman had originally obtained his seniority. The argument for this maneuver was that such offers were justified in that the second injury had occurred while the employee had been operating in a lower grade job (which, however, had also been a lighter job). When the employee and a Union official responded that such work was inappropriate and out of keeping with medical reports, a conflict broke out between the Union and W.C.B. officials versus company officials, each side accusing the other of bad faith. There were further delays as the Company referred the matter to higher management, and a full 6 months passed with the patient in limbo despite having been pronounced fit for work by the rehabilitation team in the Pain Clinic, and without the medical office of the Company disputing that the man was indeed fit for work.

It is easy to see from this kind of interaction how easy it may be for an individual to remain locked in an adversary position, angry and confused, and how he might be baited to contribute to his downfall by behaving in an irrational or angry way. One might also see how the politics of the situation can become so complicated that company officials might sincerely perceive themselves as being victimized and bullied by injured workmen and their agency allies.

A meeting finally was called between senior plant and personnel officials, members of the Union, Workmen's Compensation Board representative and staff of the Pain Clinic. Accusations of bad faith were again traded. On the one side there was the innuendo that this employee was like all other poor risk employees. From the other side came the charge that several appropriate jobs for which the employee had skills and seniority had been assigned to other workmen in that employee's old section in the 6 months since the application had been made for him to return to work. In what was obviously a stand-off, the threat was finally made by the Union officer that the matter would soon be brought before the courts. Meanwhile, the "rehabilitated" patient was now beginning again to telephone the Pain Clinic, complaining of depression and feelings that he was going to lose control, complaining of aggravation of his pain and renewed family distress, and it was evident that his morale was down to the point where emergency psychological intervention had to be mounted. The patient was saying, "At this point, if the Company were to call me to go into work today, I don't think I would last the day."

It is worth considering the incentives and disincentives at the employee's and employer's side for any change to be admitted. For the employee a number of obstacles may be put in his way as he attempts to resume his occupation. These obstacles combined with his loss of morale and continued chronic discomfort may outweigh any hopes for return to work, and the easier course may be to renew the complaint, reaffirm the disability and accept the consequences of chronic invalid status, small pension, and adjustment of family and environment to his disabled posture. On the employer's side, the number of injured employees registered against the company is disadvantageous both in terms of lost man-hours and in terms of compensation board assessments, so that, in general, rehabilitation or preventative programs are an asset to the companies. When the companies are dealing with single individuals, however, and particularly if the company is large, the contradictory principle also holds—that, in general, individuals who have been sick and off work are as a rule more likely to be a liability in the future than are employees with no such record. The working place itself may also be hostile to the return of an injured individual because such a return displaces workmen who had temporarily assumed the vacated position and imposes a liability on foremen and junior management. It is further worth noting that the return of someone to the work place may be through the channel of Workmen's Compensation Board intervention which involves some aspect of "vested interest" or through the channel of Union intervention which involves some aspects of adversary relationship. As a result of this, the transition of injured workman from chronic invalid to productive workman is hampered.

Fortunately in this case, a few weeks after court action was threatened by the Union the workman was suddenly returned to his original job, original classification and appropriate pay scale. Follow-up 6 months later revealed that there was no further serious pain complaint, psychological disturbance, family disruption, or conflictual relationship.

Although this case history is dramatic, it is not atypical and is brought forward to illustrate that the matter of medical treatment and rehabilitation must be considered within a much larger frame of reference than that of pathophysiology or psychological distress. Formulations such as "compensation neurosis" are woefully inadequate, and there is much more to rehabilitation than doing a good job at the Rehabilitation Center.

The authors wish to add that it is not their intention to vilify employers or agencies any more than it is their intention to label injured workmen as "unmotivated." In fact, many companies are taking a very enlightened view of health and rehabilitation in the work place and have given a great deal of latitude to their medical departments to develop positive, realistic and sensitive programs to assist the employees, in both preventative and remedial aspects. Management in some companies also takes a very responsible attitude toward creating conditions that avoid the difficulties that are illustrated in this case. Workmen's Compensation Boards also have frequently been the object of attack. They do, however, what they are legislated to do and their critics have not been prolific in describing workable alternatives to current systems.

Application to Rehabilitation Practice

This chapter raises issues. It does not make understanding of the occupational role and chronic disability simple because it is not simple. In devising strategy for intervention, the problem must be formulated in a way which comprehends the levels at which change is simultaneously occurring. One may choose to divide the problem into "biological," "psychological," and "social" aspects and to base intervention on the tripartite formulation. Relevant biological variables have to include a description of what is reversible and at what price. Where chronicity of some aspects of the problem are to be expected, this must be defined along with a description of what accommodations are apt to be most adaptive and stable. Consideration of the psychological dimension involves description of the affective state and the cognitions and evaluations that the patient brings to bear in interpreting his problem. Relevant here is personality structure, available adaptive repertoire, and intellectual capacity. The social dimension includes assessment of the resources on which the individual may draw, description of family role functions, the nature of the occupational role and intervening illness role, and the relationship of these things to the interfaces of medical service, agency, employer, peer, etc.

In rehabilitation, no unitary intervention can be considered sufficient. Protected situations must be provided in which lost occupational role behaviors and damaged familial roles may be restored and mastery once again be experienced. As this occurs within the rehabilitation agency framework, communications must simultaneously be maintained with external agencies and important other elements in the prospective worker's ecology. Resolution of the chronic disability and reassumption of the occupational role involve much more than medical rehabilitation, or even vocational rehabilitation practice, and in the final analysis enter the fields of politics and big economy.

REFERENCES

1. CALLAHAN, E. M., CARROLL, S., REVIER, P., GRILHONLEY, E., AND DUNN, D. The sick role in chronic illness: Some restrictions. *J. Chron. Dis.*, *19:* 883–897, 1966.
2. DEUTCH, C. P. Family factors in the home adjustment of the severely disabled. *Marriage and Family Living*, *22:* 312–316, 1962.
3. ENGEL, G. Psychogenic pain and the pain prone patient. *Am. J. Med.*, *54:* 899–918, 1959.
4. FORDYCE, W. Operant conditioning in the treatment of chronic pain. *Arch. Phys. Med. Rehabil.*, *54:* 399–408, 1973.
5. GALLAGHER, E. B. Lines of reconstruction and extension in the Parsonian sociology of illness. In *Patients, Physicians and Illness*, Ed. 3, edited by E. G. Jalo. Free Press, New York, 1979.
6. HEARD, C. Occupational role acquisition. *Am. J. Occupat. Ther.*, *31:* 243–247, 1977.
7. MECHANIC, D. Stress, illness and illness behaviour. *J. Human Stress*, *3:* 2–6, 1976.
8. PILOWSKY, I., AND SPENCE, N. Pain and illness behaviour: A comparative study. *J. Psychol. Res.*, *20:* 131–134, 1975.
9. PILOWSKY, I. Abnormal illness behaviour. *Br. J. Med. Psychiatr.*, *42:* 347–351, 1969.
10. SERES, J. AND NEWMAN, R. I. Results of treatment of chronic low back pain at the Portland Pain Centre. *J. Neurosurg.*, *45:* 32–36, 1976.
11. SHEALY, N. *The Pain Game.* Celestial Acts Press, Millbank, CA, 1976.
12. STERNBACH, R. *Pain Patients—Traits and Treatment.* Academic Press, New York, 1974.
13. STERNBACH, R. Chronic low back pain: The low back loser. *Postgrad. Med.*, *53:* 135–138, 1973.
14. SWANSON, D. W., FLOSECH, A. C., AND SWENSON, W. M. Programs for managing chronic pain: I and II. *Mayo Clin. Proc.*, *51:* 401–411, 1976.
15. SZASZ, T. The nature of pain. *Arch. Neurol. Psychiatr.*, *74:* 174–181, 1955.
16. SZASZ, T. *Pain and Pleasure: A Study of Bodily Feelings.* Tavistock Publications, London, 1957.
17. WARING, E. M., MOHAMED, S. N., BOYD, D. B., AND WEISZ, G. Chronic Pain and The Family: A Review. Presented at the Second World Congress of the International Association for the Study of Pain (IASP), Montreal, Canada, August 1978.
18. WOODFORDE, J. AND MERSKEY, H. Personality traits of patients with chronic pain. *J. Psychosom. Res.*, *16:* 167–172, 1972.

6

Women with Chronic Pain

JOAN CROOK, R.N.

Here in a grotto, shelter'd close from air,
and screen'd in shades from days' detested glare,
She sighs forever on her pensive bed,
Pain at her side, and Megrim at her head.

Alexander Pope (21)

I noted she was rather high strung and Elavil 25 milligrams 3 times a day may help her symptoms.

She complains bitterly of pain and her complaints are really quite expressive. I think she rather enjoys her disability status right now.

These two statements, extracted from the charts of female patients referred to a University Pain Clinic, suggest certain images, attitudes, and emotional responses. Similarly, a group of women discussing their initial experiences with pain noted the interpretations they were given:

A tall girl is going to have back pain.

The same doctor, who told me I had a low tolerance level, had gone through 3 days of labor with me 2 years before and should have known what I could take.

There are many unquestioned attitudes of health professionals toward their female patients and unexamined expectations of patients toward health professionals, particularly physicians—unexamined and unquestioned perhaps because they are so familiar. As Chomsky (2) observed, it is all too easy for the familiar to be transformed into the "natural."

One of the problems in dealing with the subject matter of this chapter is that the 'women's issue' has become a popular, familiar issue of the day. Women's issues can be easily dismissed as misplaced altruism, radical feminism, assumed to be too obvious or thoughtlessly endorsed. Nevertheless, this chapter has come to be written through the impetus arising from issues of human suffering as they apply to women. It is interesting that most of the literature on chronic pain seems to focus on men. This may be appropriate since representation in Workmen's Compensation programs and rehabilitation services involves high proportions of males. But what about the female proportion of the population who use clinic and rehabilitation services? It would be correct to say that women suffering from chronic pain face different personal, social, and cultural adjustments than do men with chronic pain. Yet, there is not a single article on women with chronic pain. It may be that it is just this area that we take so much for granted that is the one, when the questions can be properly posed, which would open up new avenues of exploration.

The purpose of this chapter is to develop the historical, social role, and socioeconomic perspectives of women with chronic pain. Historical-cultural mythology accepts female frailty as natural and, therefore, women ought to bear with it. Simultaneously, female intrusions into the work force are considered unsalutary and are done without exemptions from nurturant roles. Medical-psychological viewpoints may perpetuate this.

Socioeconomically, disparities exist and persevere in the rehabilitation and insurance industries. These tend to favor the return of women to the kitchen or, if without family support, to penury and the return of the working women to the job ghettos.

Historical Perspectives

One way to understand the current occupational and illness behavior of women is to consider the historical and philosophical origins of present attitudes and beliefs.

The biologically oriented concept of illness in women has its ancient history in the annals of medicine; its treatment in the medical literature of the 19th century has been extensively reviewed (1, 6, 7, 24). The argument of the time was that women's normal state was to be sick, and the source of all their troubles was found directly in their vulnerable reproductive system. This was advanced not as empirical observation but presumed to be physiological fact. Each cycle throughout women's reproductive life demanded varying periods of confinement, invalidism and indisposition. Further, as Smith-Rosenberg and Rosenberg (24) note: "Nurturance, intuitive morality, domesticity, passivity, and affection" were women's ideal social characteristics, and these were assumed to have "a deeply rooted biological basis." These same authors suggest that the biological image granted women was consistent with their traditional social role, and it served the purpose of eliminating two of the threats to traditional role definition: demands by women for higher education and birth control. As their article (24) demonstrates, the sociocultural context not only affects the interpretation of symptoms but also conditions the responses that are identified to deal with the problem, i.e., the "treatments" which are defined as most appropriate, and, more importantly, maintains traditional social values and roles.

The counterpart of the biological version of women's frailty is found in the history of hysteria (3, 6, 7, 13, 16, 23). Although the concept of hysteria has changed over time, hysteria has always been viewed as a "female" experience and one which has almost always carried with it a pejorative implication.

The hysterical female is described in the predominantly male literature of the 19th century by Smith-Rosenberg (23) as a "child-woman, highly impressionable, labile, superficially sexual, exhibitionistic, given to dramatic body language and grand gesture, with strong dependency needs and decided ego weaknesses." The author notes that these characteristics were the same traits and behaviors into which female children were socialized.

Hysteria was the impetus to Freud's totally new "scientific" approach to the medical management of women (16, 18). The Freudian theory of female nature held that women were still sick and their sickness continued to be predestined by their anatomy, but this time due to the absence of a penis rather than the pressure of a "domineering" uterus.

Nevertheless, 19-century women were not merely passive victims of medical science. Since all roles serve important functions—allowing satisfaction and mastery, and preserving self-esteem—women were able to turn their sick roles to their own advantage. Some women resorted to sickness as a means of birth and sex control; others, as a means of gaining attention and a limited amount of power in their families; still others, to gain certain exemptions from social obligations, to be protected and provided for economically. These satisfactions were short-lived, and the sick-role exemptions placed women into increasingly intolerable social roles as they were denied access to education, productive activity outside the home, and safe birth control.

As hysteria came to be identified as a 'functional' disease and therefore not a 'real' disease, hysterical women, in some sense, began to be regarded as frauds. Not surprisingly, a sense of superiority and hostility permeated most physicians' writings as they viewed the "nervous" female as being innately weak, possessed by a childlike incompetence, and possibly manipulative (23–25).

These historical heritages continue to impose themselves in concepts, language, and application of present-day medicine as it relates to women in general and, more specifically, to women in pain. They most often express themselves in the mind-body dichotomy. Pain patients, as Tunks (26) observed, "find themselves caught in a dualistic mode of thinking which splits off the psychological and social from what is demonstrably physical." They are labeled, usually pejoratively, using such terms as "compensation neurosis," "psychogenic pain," and the like. When the pain patient is female, additional labels are preferentially introduced, i.e., "fragile," "hysterical," "dependent," "neurotic," and "passive."

HISTORICAL INFLUENCES TODAY

Explanations based on the assumption of the frailty of the female body and its "problems" throughout the female life cycle often are the first explanations given to women complaining of pain. Mary, at 21, was told "women generally have a low tolerance to pain"; at 46, it was suggested to Pauline that she was going through the change of life. Their physicians suggested rest, confinement to bed for varying periods of time, curtailing or discontinuing physical activities and work, and, in general, limiting any activities which caused discomfort. One could appreciate a physician's choice of conservative management of symptoms in each of these examples, but the choice of explanation did nothing to allay fears but rather reinforced helplessness.

Women with chronic pain are often offered psychological explanations. Although men with chronic pain suffer similarly from psychological reductionism, women suffer a double liability in this regard. As a recent example, Lennane and Lennane (13) examined how medicine defines, researches, and organizes the management of disorders that affect women. In an examination of primary dysmenorrhea, nausea in pregnancy, pain in labor, and infantile behavior disorders (colic), the authors argue that despite the well-documented presence of organic etiological factors the medical literature is characterized by an unjustifiably simplistic recourse to psychogenesis and a correspondingly inadequate, even derisive, approach to their management. Health professionals are more likely to offer psychotherapy and psychotherapeutic drugs to women and are more willing to label women as hysterical (4, 9, 10). Furthermore, women are more likely to interpret symptoms psychologically, and present them in this way, and are more likely to accept psychological interpretations and treatments (1, 10).

Splitting interpretations of pain into exclusive biological and psychological categories tends to be a powerful means of placing the blame on the patient. Patients who are made to feel they have, albeit unwittingly, caused the pain are also made to feel they deserve it. "You know that the pain hurts and the doctors are telling you that it's because you haven't come to grips with it. They almost assume that you want to stay this way, that you are 'resisting' giving it up."

Even family and friends contribute to helping the patient feel morally responsible for the pain. "My friend, after asking if there was anything she could do to help me, said, 'I can't afford to get sick; I can't give myself the luxury'." But the woman in pain also shares this double standard, for as Janet responded, "I was the one to say to myself 'I can't get sick. Who will take care of my children'?"

Nevertheless, the patients in the group were aware of the potential misuse of their pain, particularly as a way of avoiding social 'obligations,' but were equally aware that family and friends were interpreting their 'excuse' as manipulative or as avoiding responsibility.

Other difficulties arise when psychological explanations of pain or disease are given to women. There is an unfortunately widespread view that the patient whose symptoms are psychogenic is not entitled to any relief: "...you will have to learn to live with it." Or the opposite is possible, that is, the patient may find herself on large doses of tranquilizers and pain killers" ...so much so you end up feeling like a junkie."

Social Role Perspectives

Central to the analysis of this chapter is the assumption that culture, social structure, and the individual are integrally linked (8, 11, 15). Roles are considered to be the major link between social structure and the individual. The power of roles is so great that it has been asserted that a person's perceptions, motivations, self-concept, and psychological function are "shaped and steered by the specific configuration of roles" incorporated from society (11).

In considering a social system, one encounters religious, familial, occupational, educational, and other systems all interrelated. There is also a complexity in the pattern of roles when considering any individual within a social system. For example, one single individual in the course of a day can demonstrate membership in social, occupational, and illness roles and within all of these have a personal self-concept (in Transactional Analysis, this is called a "script"). A person's role is reciprocal to the roles held by others. It should also be evident that there are a variety of roles an individual may hold within a single role system.

The difference between male and female roles is of particular importance. It would be correct to say that family and caretaking roles are much more specifically bound to the female than they are to the male. The women who were seen in discussion groups felt that one of their primary functions was to maintain the interior life and emotional climate of the family and its environment. Although it has been suggested that women's roles are reltively undemanding and, therefore, they have ample time to be sick or have pain, these women felt that their caretaking responsibilities made their disability very disturbing to family equilibrium (20).

The socialization of women to serve others within their nurturant role is an important determinant of how they perceive the world and how they attempt to maintain adequacy of role function (17). In pain rehabilitation, it is often this issue that surfaces with so-called resistance to change or noncompliance. Janet provides a good example: She never seemed to find the time to practice her relaxation exercises between biofeedback sessions. When this was pointed out to her, after clarifying the expectations, Janet said she felt guilty leaving all the work just to spend time on herself. "You don't want your kids or husband to do all your work."

When female pain patients can no longer participate in physical activities with family and friends, it becomes a very basic threat and it needs to be resolved, as one of our patients said: "I used to feel sorry for my kids and husband ending up with me, but then I discovered that they didn't love me just for jogging around the block with them. I learned that there are other ways of togetherness for families and friends. Mentally and emotionally we are much closer now."

The caring and doing for others becomes a part of a complex of expectations of others. Some women, realizing that they could not keep up and could not renegotiate relationships on a different basis, experienced loss of relationships. "You begin to see the transformation in people. They get tired of seeing you sick all the time." Loss of relationships tends to isolate the women even further; such losses are often a basic threat to their role identity, producing anxiety and very often guilt. What seem to be obvious solutions to health professionals—for example, going off for a weekend by oneself or placing a severely handicapped mother in a nursing home—are not such easy solutions for the woman.

Illness roles may be differently perceived in the case of women as compared with men. In general, the illness role involves exemptions for anyone who is ill. The female role in illness may be diverse, in that exemption from family caretaking duties does not occur as readily as for men. It is more commonly encountered, more socially acceptable, for a man to abandon his family responsibilities on account of sickness or occupational pressures than for a woman to do the same thing. The modification of roles during illness is complicated by factors of chronicity (see Chapter 4, by Gallagher and Wrobel). Women's help-seeking behavior also appears to vary, depending on the availability of immediate social supports: for example, a mother or sister who would be available to replace them in their family roles—a role-substitution not easily accomplished (20).

What emerges from these observations is that there may be an inherent conflict between a woman in her illness role and in her other roles. Although she may be sick, she is not able to relinquish her caretaking responsibilities. This becomes more acute if there is also an occupational role. A woman has historically been seen as having invaded the working milieu, and there may be serious conflict between maintaining working capacity and maintaining a caretaker role while having an illness complaint. The tendency of social pressures and expectations are such that they would return the woman to the family role and out of the occupational role, albeit still sick.

Rosalina is an appropriate example to illustrate this point: She was "doing it all." Her Italian husband had chronic neck and back pain as the result of a work injury. He had been engaged for several years in virtually no productive activity except for frequent visits to physicians. After his injury, Rosalina had gone to work as an unskilled laborer in the textile industry at minimum wage, poor benefits and equally poor working conditions. When Rosalina was interviewed, it was apparent that they were in great financial distress but, equally important, her husband was not carrying out any paternal role with the children. She complained of 'nerves and pain' attributed to his illness. "Please get him well quick or I will lose my job." She could not carry occupational, financial and family demands productively single-handedly. She saw two choices—to return only to her homemaker, caretaker role or return to work, with the likelihood she would 'break down.' So strongly internalized was her personal caretaking role 'script' that neither she nor her husband could examine the option of her husband assuming the caretaker, homemaker role so that she could fulfill the worker 'breadwinner' role.

Socioeconomic Perspectives

In the previous sections, historical and social role perspectives were examined in relation to attitudes regarding disease and social behavior. Particular reference was made to the position in which women find themselves. The correlates of this in the social system are expressed in socioeconomic terms and can be examined in relation to rehabilitation, retraining services, and disability insurance.

Although there are no data available specifically on women with chronic pain, examining rehabilitation service areas in relation to the working woman can give us some insight into some of the services affecting women with chronic pain. Women comprise 51% of the population and 40% of the work force (5). As women continue to increase their participation in the labor force and enter a wider range of occupations, more of them will be affected by the operation of Workmen's Compensation Boards, disability insurance, rehabilitation, and retraining programs.

It has been suggested that the long-term consequences of worker injury may be more severe for women than for men (14). The reasons noted are that women tend to be more marginal workers, with less consistent work histories, lower pay, and lower ranking positions. Therefore, they are more likely to suffer uncompensated wage loss, less likely to receive rehabilitation services (12), and, with comparable levels of physical impairment, are less likely to be employed (22).

Makaruskka (14) notes that women do not appear in Worker's Compensation population in proportion to their representation in the labor force and that 5 years after injury women are less likely to be working than are the men in her samples.

Likewise, in a Canadian report prepared for the Status of Women Advisory Council, the underrepresentation of women in training programs in 1978–1979 was identified, with women comprising 45% of the unemployed but comprising only one third of the institutional training programs (5).

A report of the Woman's Bureau, Labor Canada, questions and challenges the rationale that insurance companies give to explain the higher premiums charged women for disability insurance (28).

What are some of the interpretations given for the disproportionate allocation and use of resources between males and females? From the above reports, the authors note: When men drop out of the work force after an injury, disability is assumed and the men claim compensation, but when women drop out, they have additional alternatives and socially acceptable roles and do not necessarily claim compensation (14). Likewise, women are supported by husbands who are the "breadwinners" and, therefore, do not need protection (the rationale of the insurance industry) or do not use what is available (28). This is one factor which explains the underrepresentation of women in rehabilitation services.

The second interpretation is that there are differences in occupational distribution, with women being in smaller establishments or more heavily concentrated in job "ghettos" (domestic and clerical) which are less likely to be covered by compensation (5, 14).

The third argument is that of female frailty, that is, women are simply sicker than men (this would tend to inflate female rates) (20). The opposite but related argument is that women are protected from potentially stressful or dangerous jobs because of their innate frailty (this would tend to deflate rates).

Each of these explanations is plausible, and examination of the data indicates that each has some truth to it.

Since women's absence from the work force after injury is related to marital status, household size, and age, Makaruskka's data (14) support the contention that women may have acceptable role alternatives but, as she points out, there is a large group of unmarried women for whom the consequences of impairment may be most severe, since they have neither the additional household wage earner of the married woman nor the potential earning power of the male counterpart.

Other Canadian and United States data support this point of view. Nagi (19), for example, noted that no disability-related benefit payment was received by more than half of the severely disabled, and three fourths of these were women, one fourth of whom were single, widowed, or divorced. Similarly, arguing against the assumption that working women do not require the protection afforded by insurance coverage, the Canadian report points out that 2,500,000 women under the age of 65 and over 15 are single, widowed, or divorced. (Canada's total population is 22,000,000.) One third of a million women who live with a spouse in a household of four have income at the poverty level, and there are many married women whose family life would be reduced to the poverty level or below if it were not for the fact that the wife was working (28).

The observation that there are differences in occupational distribution, with women more heavily concentrated in service or clerical areas, is unquestionably true for both Canada and the United States. Nevertheless, to continue to stream women into traditional female occupations in retraining programs not only reinforces job "ghettoization" but also prepares women for redundancy as these areas are increasingly being taken over by technological innovations (5). Likewise, these same "female" occupations have lower pay and, if compensation benefits are set at a percentage of the weekly wage as they are in some states and provinces, the inequity of payment in the labor market may be permanently built into any continuing compensation that women may secure for their expected wage loss after injury (14).

The argument of the frailty of the female has also come under criticism through an examination of mortality and morbidity data. The differences in female and male life expectancy at birth had increased to 7 years by the 1970s in Canada in favor of women (28). The limited morbidity data available in Canada show that with regard to long-term illness and disability, the rate for men is 8% higher than the rate for women (28). Morbidity data relating to incidence of illness as reported by hospitals show the male rate is higher for the most severely disabling conditions.

The morbidity data available from the United States National Health Survey in 1972 show a different picture than that of Canada. Women have higher rates than men for almost all indices of morbidity and utilization (20, 27). Several explanations have been suggested for these sex differences. Nathanson (20), for example, summarizes three possible reasons:

1. Women report more illness than men report because it is culturally more acceptable for women to be ill.
2. The sick role is more compatable with women's other role responsibilities.
3. Women have more illness because their assigned social roles are more stressful.

Verbrugge (27) provides evidence that excess female morbidity is due primarily to social and psychological factors, namely, interview behavior and illness behavior, and not to acquired or inherited health risks. The reasons for excess female morbidity have not been fully established. Nevertheless, it does not seem plausible to accept innate female frailty as the simple answer. This issue would be more clearly resolved if further efforts were directed toward examining illness behavior as a function of role socialization, role conflict arising from other role obligations, and personal role "scripts."

The observations that emerge from these data, when considered in the context of women's historical heritage and their present-day social role, suggest that women are more likely to remain at a poor level of functioning, being rather powerless to climb out of a disabled position, retreating to the home, supported by someone else, or, if unattached, relegated to poverty. Many of the benefits women receive reinforce "ghettoization," either by not being offered the same opportunity for rehabilitation or insurance services (scarce resources saved for the male "breadwinner") or being offered programs that continue to streamline women into homemaking, crafts, or clerical areas.

Summary

Hopefully, within a few years this chapter will be outdated, as it is recognized that there has been and will be change. Nevertheless, we cannot ignore the complexities that are introduced by the transition in which women presently find themselves. It will continue to be important when working with women with chronic pain to examine their social system, major occupational and familial roles, as well as their personal "script" and that of their husbands. Our own values as health professionals toward women will, if necessary, need to be reexamined within this ever-changing scene.

It is unlikely that women with chronic pain will seek or demand different services that might be more appropriate to their needs. Women are not victims of the system but, as participants, are frequently left with the unfortunate consequences of it.

As health professionals involved in the delivery of health services, participating in long-range planning or being responsible for policymaking regarding the distribution of scarce rehabilitation resources, we can facilitate change by taking every opportunity to point out that women have particular needs that are not being met, largely because of unexamined assumptions regarding what these needs are.

REFERENCES

1. CHESLER, P. *Women and Madness.* Avon Books, New York, 1972.
2. CHOMSKY, N. *Language and Mind.* Harcourt Brace Jovanovich, New York, 1968.
3. CLEGHORN, R. A. Hysteria: Multiple manifestations of semantic confusion. *Can. Psychiatr. Assoc. J., 14(6):* 539–567, 1969.
4. COOPERSTOCK, R. Psychotropic drug use among women. *Can. Med. Assoc. J., 115:* 760–763, 1976.
5. DALE, P. Women and Jobs: The Impact of Federal Government Employment Strategies on Women. Report commissioned by the Canadian Advisory Committee on the Status of Women, 1980.
6. EHRENREICH, B., AND ENGLISH, D. *For Her Own Good: 150 Years of the Experts' Advice to Women.* Anchor Press/Doubleday, New York, 1979.
7. DREIFUS, C. (Eds.) *Seizing Our Bodies: The Politics of Women's Health.* Vintage Books, New York, 1978.
8. ENGEL, G. The clinical application of the biopsychosocial model. *Am. J. Psychiatry, 137:* 535–544, 1980.
9. FRANK, J., GLIEDMAN, L. H., IMBER, S. D., NASH, E. H., AND STONE, A. R. Why patients leave psychotherapy. *A.M.A. Arch. Neurol. Psychiatry, 77:* 283–299, 1957.
10. FUNKS, V., AND BURTLE, V. (Eds.) *Women in Therapy: New Psychotherapies for a Changing Society.* Brunner/Mazel Publishers, New York, 1974.
11. GERTH, H., AND MILLS, C. W. *Character and Social Structure.* Harcourt Brace and World, New York, 1953.
12. JAFFE, A. J., DAZ, L. H., AND ADAMS, W. *Disabled Workers in the Labor Market.* Bedminster Press, New York, 1964.
13. LENNANE, K. J., AND LENNANE, R. J. Alleged psychogenic disorders in women: A possible manifestation of sexual prejudice. *N. Engl. J. Med., 288:* 288–292, 1973.
14. MAKARUSKKA, J. L. Workers' Compensation: The Long-Term Consequences of Work-Related Injury for Women. *Proceedings, Conference on Woman and the Workplace,*

Society for Occupational and Environmental Health, Washington, D. C., April 1977, pp. 293–301.

15. MECHANIC, D. *Medical Sociology: A Selective View*. Free Press, New York, 1968.
16. MERSKEY, H. *The Analysis of Hysteria*. Ballière Tindall, London, 1979.
17. MILLER, J. B. *Toward a New Psychology of Women*. Beacon Press, Boston, 1976.
18. MITCHELL, J. *Psychoanalysis and Feminism*. Vintage Books, New York, 1975.
19. NAGI, S. Z. *Disability and Rehabilitation: Legal, Clinical, and Self-Concepts and Measurement*. Ohio State University Press, Columbus, 1969.
20. NATHANSON, C. A. Illness and the feminine role: A theoretical review. *Soc. Sci. Med.*, *9:* 57–62, 1975.
21. POPE, A. The Rape of the Lock 1714. In *The Oxford Dictionary of Quotations*, Ed. 3. Oxford University Press, Oxford, 1979.
22. SAFILIOS-ROTHSCHILD, C. *The Sociology and Social Psychology of Disability and Rehabilitation*. Random House, New York, 1970.
23. SMITH-ROSENBERG, C. The hysterical woman: Sex roles and role conflict in 19th century America. *Soc. Res.*, *39:* 652–678, 1972.
24. SMITH-ROSENBERG, C., AND ROSENBERG, C. The female animal: Medical and biological views of woman and her role in 19th century America. *J. Am. History*, *60:* 332–356, 1973.
25. SPANOS, N. P., AND GOTTLIEB, J. Demonic possession, mesmerism and hysteria: A social psychological perspective on their historical interrelations. *J. Abnorm. Psychol.*, *88(5):* 527–546, 1978.
26. TUNKS, E. A client centered approach to rehabilitation of patients with chronic pain. Paper presented at 2nd World Congress of ISAP, Montreal, Quebec, August 31, 1978.
27. VERBRUGGE, L. M. Females and illness: Recent trends in sex differences in the United States. *J. Health Soc. Behav.*, *17:* 387–403, 1976.
28. Woman's Bureau 74, Labor Canada. Time to Reform Traditional Insurance Practices to Eliminate Sex Discrimination. Presented at a meeting of Management, Manufacturers Life Insurance Co., Toronto, November 12, 1974, pp. 99–106.

7

Behavior and Cognitive Therapies

ROY CAMERON, Ph.D.

Behavioral Treatments for Chronic Pain

The objective of this chapter is to provide a critical overview of behavioral approaches to the treatment of chronic pain. An attempt has been made to provide a comprehensive review, although space limitations preclude an exhaustive coverage of the literature. The focus is on research relevant to clinical decision making; studies conducted with clinical populations are emphasized. Behavioral approaches may be classified as operant, biofeedback or cognitive behavioral skill training. The chapter will consider each of these approaches in turn.

OPERANT TREATMENT

Chronic pain problems are sometimes analyzed and treated using an operant conditioning framework. This approach was pioneered by Wilbert Fordyce and his colleagues. The basic principles underlying the operant model have been summarized by Fowler et al. (31, p. 1226):

1. Behavior is largely a function of its consequences.
2. Behavior which is followed by positive or rewarding consequences will tend to be maintained or to increase in rate.
3. Behavior which is followed by neutral consequences will tend to diminish or drop out altogether.

These principles suggest that if behaviors signalling pain result in positive consequences, these "pain behaviors" will increase in frequency. Common pain behaviors include verbal pain complaints, wincing, moaning, rubbing affected areas, taking medications, avoiding activities associated with pain, reclining and seeking medical attention. The patient may receive attention (often sympathetic attention) and frequently is relieved of responsibilities when such behaviors are emitted. Attention and legitimized abdication of responsibility are presumably rewarding experiences for many people. To the extent that pain behavior leads to such rewards, the frequency of the pain behaviors may be increased or maintained by a process of operant conditioning. Thus, pain behavior originally elicited by organic factors may come to occur, totally or in part, in response to reinforcing environmental events.

It should be emphasized that proponents of operant treatment do not suggest that the process described above is conscious or deliberately manipulative. It is assumed that pain patients are probably experiencing genuine subjective distress even when their behavior is being reinforced by environmental consequences (as the subjective distress many of us experience at the sight of blood is real, although presumably learned). In commenting on this issue, Finneson (24) has reported that patients believed to have a significant operant component to their pain, and initially suspected of being malingerers, were observed surreptitiously and found to continue to show evidence of disability even when they were not aware they were being observed.

Some experimental evidence confirms that pain behavior may be influenced considerably by environmental factors. For instance, Wooley et al. (82) have described a study in which chronic pain patients were asked to immerse their hands in ice water in a laboratory situation. In one condition, an attempt was made to have the patient-subject perceive the experimenter as someone who was sympathetic and prepared to reinforce pain behavior. In a second case, there was a suggestion that pain tolerance and coping would be rewarded. On average, subjects (Ss) in the first group withdrew their arms (pain behavior) after 74 sec. vs. 320 sec. in the second group. Only one S in the first group endured the full 360 sec. trial vs. 9 of 12 who tolerated the full trial in the second condition. Fordyce (28) also has described some interesting experimental studies which suggest that factors other than aversive physical sensations may influence pain behavior.

An operant analysis of chronic pain behavior suggests two intervention strategies. First, the model predicts that environmentally controlled pain behaviors will decrease in frequency if reinforcing consequences are withheld. Second, the patient's functional status will improve if "well behaviors," which are incompatible with pain behaviors, are rewarded. (It is sometimes necessary not only to reinforce but also to train adaptive behaviors if these are not in the patient's repertoire.) Operant programs described in the literature have been conducted on an inpatient basis. However, it also seems important to attempt to alter the patient's normal environment in order to increase the probability that healthy behaviors will continue to be reinforced and that pain behaviors will not be reinforced after the patient is discharged. This is generally done by training family members in the use of operant principles (25–27).

Common reinforcers of pain behavior are social attention and analgesic medication (which serves as a negative reinforcer by reducing pain). During treatment, attention is withheld when patients manifest typical pain behaviors. However, acute distress and indications that the patient requires relief or assistance are, of course, responded to. Medication is not administered contingent upon pain: rather, it is provided at fixed intervals. Usually the amount of medication is gradually reduced during the course of treatment. The patient's medications are mixed in a flavored syrup to form a "pain cocktail" that allows the medications to be reduced without the patient's awareness (although the patient may know in advance what is planned and agree to the gradual tapering of medication).

The process of withholding social attention in an attempt to extinguish pain behaviors must be handled delicately. The therapist must walk a narrow line which involves being firm, yet not appearing to be callous. Wooley et al. (82) have provided a list of common patient behaviors and possible therapist responses which provides some useful clinical guidelines. For example, for the patient behavior of "dividing staff," counterproductive responses might include the sympathetic response of "advocacy" or a more directive response of "clarification." In such a case, the authors would suggest referring the problem back to the patient and one primary therapist. In a similar manner, suggestions are given for management of helpless behavior, demands, compliance, veiled hostility, etc.

At the same time the pain behaviors are being extinguished, healthy behavior is reinforced. While effective reinforcers must be identified on an individual basis for each patient (e.g., one may thoroughly enjoy attention, while another avoids attention), commonly used reinforcers are rest and social attention. Fordyce (27) has emphasized that social reinforcement for well behavior may be especially critical during the time it is being withheld from pain behavior: unless the patient receives a reasonable level of staff attention he is likely to feel that he is being poorly treated by an indifferent staff.

One of the most commonly reinforced well behaviors is exercise. The patient who is exercising is not only engaging in well behavior per se but also developing strength and endurance which will make it possible to engage in a wider range of normal activities. Typically, the exercise program begins at a level somewhat below the patient's demonstrated capacity so that success and encouragement are possible from the outset. The exercise quota is gradually raised, and reinforcement is withheld until the quota has been met.

The most detailed description of operant clinical methods is to be found in Fordyce's (27) recent book. This is a valuable reference work for clinicians working with chronic pain patients.

Inpatient treatment of the sort just described lasts about 3 weeks in some settings (70) and, not uncommonly, 2 months in others (2). Clearly, it is a very expensive form of treatment for patients and staff. Nonetheless, given the enormous personal and social costs of chronic pain and disability, it might be cost efficient if it is effective.

How effective, then, is the treatment? Published reports are now available describing treatment results in at least six settings. These include the Mayo Clinic (53, 74–76), Rancho Los Amigos Hospital (14, 15), the Portland Pain Center (70), the San Diego V.A. Hospital (36, 41, 72), the University of Minnesota (2) and the University of Washington (29, 30). In addition, Wooley et al. (82) have described the results of a similar program for a more heterogeneous group of chronic illness patients.

Many of these programs include a wide variety of interventions (such as individual therapy, group therapy, biofeedback and vocational counselling) in addition to the operant program. It is not possible to unequivocally attribute any posttreatment improvement which may be observed following such programs to operant treatment per se. The programs which appear to be most purely operant in orientation are those of Fordyce et al. (30), Cairns and his colleagues (14, 15), and Anderson et al. (2).

Fordyce et al. (30) report on 36 patients treated over a 3½-year period. This study will be described in some detail to convey an impression of the nature and results of such programs. The research is an uncontrolled treatment outcome study. The participants appear to have been difficult cases: on an average they had had pain for 92.7 months and had had 2.7 major operations for pain. The modal medical diagnosis was "mechanical back pain." The patients were selected as being reasonable candidates for operant treatment (e.g., there was evidence of operant pain, they seemed responsive to reinforcers controllable in the hospital setting).

Inpatient treatment lasted from 4 to 12 weeks, with some patients receiving additional outpatient treatment for up to 24 weeks. Treatment was tailored to the specific needs of the patient. For instance, if employment was the objective, the patient was assigned to a related job station during treatment and was assisted in finding suitable work or vocational training at the end of the program. If the goal was socialization, socializing activities were developed and encouraged. In most cases, spouses attended training sessions held twice weekly. Daily activity diaries were maintained by the patients. Operant treatment and medication management were conducted as described previously.

Pretreatment, posttreatment (at the end of the inpatient phase) and follow-up assessments (an average of 22 months after treatment ended) were conducted. There was a significant increase in "uptime" (i.e., not reclining). The mean weekly uptime rose from 64.0 hr during the preadmission week and 59.2 hr during the first admission week to 88.9 hr at the end of treatment and 94.9 hr at follow-up. These data suggest that uptime increased approximately 50% on average with treatment. Exercise tolerance also increased between the beginning and the end of treatment among patients in the various exercise programs: daily walking distance more than doubled (to over one mile on average), while number of sit-ups and number of rows woven in occupational therapy approximately doubled. Fordyce et al. (30) note that these exercise increases, all of which are statistically significant, are actually underestimates of the patients' posttreatment exercise tolerance since quotas were not raised after a given patient had attained a level of performance deemed adequate for treatment purposes. Medication use dropped dramatically by the end of inpatient treatment: use of analgesic medication (narcotic and nonnarcotic) dropped to very low levels—approximately one sixth of pretreatment levels; use of sedatives and hypnotics dropped somewhat as well. As the authors point out, the fact that use of medication decreased means that increases in uptime and exercise tolerance cannot be attributed to masking effects of drugs. Over 50% of patients failed to provide information on medication use at follow-up, and the authors interpret this omission rate as implying that relapse may have occurred after discharge. At follow-up patients were asked to rate on a 10-point scale (10 = maximum pain) the amount of pain they remembered having at admission and discharge as well as their current pain level. Average ratings were 8.6 at admission, 6.0 at discharge and 6.2 at follow-up. Although patients reported still having substantial pain at discharge and follow-up, the ratings suggested there had been a statistically significant decrease over the course of treatment, which was maintained at follow-up.

There are a number of methodological limitations which create difficulties in interpreting these findings. No control groups were included in the study. Hence it is not possible to determine what proportion of the treatment gains are attributable to the specific contribution of operant conditioning (vs. physiotherapy, vocational therapy, nonspecific demand characteristic effects, etc.). Candidates were screened by a physiatrist (who looked for discrepancies between pain behavior and organic pathology), a psychologist and, sometimes, a social worker (both of the latter explored relationships between pain behavior and reinforcing consequences): no information is provided about the number of patients screened out, so it is difficult to know if the sample was typical of chronic pain patients. Follow-up data were gathered by questionnaire, and questions may be raised about the reliability and validity of these data. Fordyce et al. (30) note that self-reported ratings of uptime during the preadmission period correlated 0.82 with average weekly uptime during the first week in hospital when the patients were under observation: they interpret this as evidence that self-report data may be accurate. However, it would seem that while patients would have no reason to distort data before treatment, they might be inclined to exaggerate improvement in self-reports after treatment, especially when they know that they will not be subsequently coming under direct observation and no check will be made on their self-reports. The validity of retrospective pain ratings, in which patients attempted to recall pain levels some 2 years earlier, is particularly dubious. Finally, it is noteworthy that many patients failed to provide follow-up data. For instance, only 17 of the original 36 provided complete information on uptime, and the follow-up estimate of uptime is based on this self-selected group. If it is assumed that failure to report completely is more likely to occur among people doing poorly, the follow-up data may overestimate the level of functioning after discharge. Many of these points have been made previously by Turk and Genest (79). Indeed, Fordyce et al. (30) themselves commented upon the methodological limitations of this important study. While the data may not show conclusively that operant treatment is effective, the results of the program appear to be very impressive given the characteristics of the sample. The results and limitations of this study are generally representative of the other studies reporting results of operant programs. It is noteworthy that the programs on which published outcome data are available tend to be located at world renowned institutions: patients often make a "pilgrimage" from some distance to get there, and presumably the treatment experience is often rather momentous. These factors may enhance treatment efficacy. One wonders whether the same program conducted in the local general hospital would be as effective.

Cairns and Pasino (14) have conducted what appears to be the only controlled evaluation of operant treatment. Nine patients were assigned to one of three experimental conditions: 1) a control group which received occupational and physical therapy comparable to experimental groups, 2) a group which received verbal reinforcement from the physical therapists for activity increases, and 3) a group which initially received graphed feedback about the day's performance posted over their beds and subsequently received verbal reinforcement from staff as well. The results indicated that there were no significant increases in activity among controls or participants in group 3 while they received graphed feedback only. Significant increases in activity were observed under the verbal reinforcement (group 2) and graph plus verbal reinforcement (group 3, second stage) conditions. This pattern of results suggests that activity levels can be increased with verbal reinforcement. After an increase in activity had been elicited through verbal reinforcement, the reinforcement was withheld (extinction) in this study. The result was a sharp drop in activity levels. The authors note that this extinction effect implies that modification of the natural environment to ensure selective reinforcement of healthy behavior is crucial for long-term clinical management.

While many of the programs listed earlier have produced what appear to be impressive results, none of them has been evaluated against a control group, except the study by Cairns and Pasino (14) which demonstrates improvement with operant treatment. However, it provides no evidence that treatment effects will be maintained upon discharge: indeed, it demonstrates that improvement is quite vulnerable to extinction even within the treatment setting. It is a very small-scale study, involving few patients and a limited number of dependent variables. Also, it is noteworthy that the authors do not (apparently) report explicitly that patients were assigned randomly to treatment conditions: it is not clear whether this represents an oversight in reporting or suggests a potential methodological problem which may undermine interpretation of the between-group comparisons. In sum, while clinical reports seem impressive, the hard evidence that operant treatment is effective is scanty at present.

Which patients might be expected to benefit from operant treatment? The first criterion is that a diagnosis of operant pain has been established. Fordyce (27) has outlined excellent detailed guidelines for conducting assessments to determine whether pain behaviors are being reinforced. The second important requirement is that the patient finds the treatment acceptable. Fordyce (27) has provided useful suggestions for presenting such programs to patients in terms which may reduce the patient's defensiveness. Swanson et al. (75) have further suggested that it may be useful to allow the patient an opportunity to observe the program before entering. They reported that 24% of their first 50 patients dropped out of the program within the first 10 days after entering (74). After they switched to a more prolonged observation period (1–2 days) which not only allowed them to collect more data on the patient but also gave the patient a chance to observe the program directly before deciding whether to enter, the attrition rate dropped to 6% (75). There is some preliminary evidence that patients with intact families derive most long-term benefit from such programs. Wooley et al. (82) found that among a sample of 12 patients, all patients deemed successful at a 1-year follow-up came from intact families (i.e., were either living with a spouse or were under 18 years of age and living at home with both parents). None of the failures came from intact families. Cross-validating evidence was found in a second study. It is not clear why patients with intact families did better. Wooley et al. (82) provided operant training for family members, so patients with intact families may have returned to more supportive natural environments after treatment. Alternatively, it may be plausible to argue that patients from intact families (i.e., patients who have established and maintained stable relationships) are more "stable" people, with more personal skills and resources; if so, they may have a better prognosis on these grounds alone. It might be noted here that while many operant programs train family members, Anderson et al. (2) have also provided behavioral counselling to the patient's family physician to help promote maintenance.

Maruta et al. (53) have identified a number of variables related to prognosis with operant treatment (blended with other modalities). The study compared patients rated successes (n = 34) vs. failures (n = 35) at a 1-year follow-up. Compared with "failure" patients, "success" patients had a shorter duration problem (average of 63.6 months vs. 105.6 months), less work time lost (average of 11.2 months vs. 31.4 months), fewer pain-related operations (average of 1.1 vs. 2.8), less dependence on medication and lower pretreatment pain reports. The authors have developed a prognostic rating scale on the basis of their findings, although, as they note, it requires cross-validation. Interestingly, these authors found that the incidence of disability compensation was *not* significantly different in the "success" and "failure" groups. However, given the small sample sizes, this finding warrants replication.

Inpatient operant treatment is logistically difficult in many settings. While outpatient treatment of this sort is possible, it is difficult. Fordyce (27) has discussed outpatient operant treatment in detail. He suggests that two strategies may be followed. One is to train family members in operant principles. The second involves training the patient to become his own change agent. There does not appear to be any data on the efficacy of such outpatient therapy.

BIOFEEDBACK THERAPY

There has been an explosion of interest in the use of biofeedback during the past 10 years. In general, biofeedback involves providing information to patients about changes in physiological functions of which there is normally no awareness. The target physiological variable is electronically monitored, and information about changes in functioning are "fed back" to the patient in the form of easily detectable signals. For instance, with EMG biofeedback, increases in muscle contraction may be signaled by an increase in the rate of auditory clicks, while decreases in tension produce a reduction in the click rate. The objective is to use such feedback to teach patients to voluntarily control physiological processes believed to be causally linked to their clinical symptoms. Clinical biofeedback applications were inspired largely by the work of Miller and his colleagues who demonstrated conditioning of visceral responses, although some of this pioneering work has proven difficult to replicate (58).

The pain syndromes for which this form of treatment has most often been employed are muscle contraction and vascular headache, although there have been reports of biofeedback being used to treat other types of pain problems as well. The use of biofeedback to treat headache, in particular, has captured the interest of clinicians and researchers. There is now an extensive and rapidly proliferating literature in this area. It would not be feasible to attempt an exhaustive review here. In any case, a number of recent comprehensive reviews are available (6, 11, 20, 43, 80).

The etiology of muscle contraction, or tension, headache is not fully understood (3). This type of head pain is believed by many experts to be related to sustained contraction of the muscles of the forehead, scalp or neck (3, 52). It has been suggested that muscle contraction headaches are triggered by psychological stress (19, 51).

Based on the evidence that there was an association between muscle contraction headache and resting levels of frontalis (forehead) EMG (66), Budzynski et al. (12) used frontalis EMG feedback to treat 5 tension headache patients. Their pioneering report indicated that during the treatment period, there was a decline in EMG levels, headache intensity and headache duration. During this treatment period, the patients were to practice at home the relaxation skills acquired during feedback sessions. Three months after treatment ended, 2 patients reported that headaches had been eliminated and 1 reported a significant reduction, while the remaining 2 patients reported that headaches returned after the end of treatment. However, both of these relapsed patients reported that they had stopped practicing relaxation exercises at home; when they resumed daily relaxation periods, both showed a reduction in headache, which lasted throughout the rest of the 3-month follow-up period. Although this was an exploratory, uncontrolled study, the treatment approach was creative and seemed to hold clinical promise. It proved to be a seminal study which spawned a great deal of interest among clinical investigators.

In general, subsequent research suggests that tension headache patients report improvement with EMG feedback. A number of studies comparing EMG feedback with no treatment or nominal treatment control groups have yielded data which offer fairly strong evidence for the effectiveness of EMG biofeedback (13, 37). As Jessup et al. (43, p. 239) have noted, such studies suggest that "the overall effects of biofeedback...cannot be dismissed as due to 'spontaneous remission,' regression toward the mean, maturational processes in the subjects, or the passage of time. A slightly broader data base...would strengthen confidence in these conclusions, assuming the new findings were congruent with reports to date."

However, a number of fundamental questions remain unanswered. First, as noted above, the treatment rationale is based on the assumption that high levels of muscle tension give rise to the pain reported. Turk et al. (80) note that the available data raise serious questions about this assumed relationship. Several studies have suggested that headache activity may be independent of elevated EMG levels and clinical improvement may be independent of EMG changes. For instance, Gray et al. (35) found EMG levels were not significantly higher during headache periods than during baseline. Holroyd et al. (39) found that EMG feedback resulted in reduced EMG but no change in headache activity; conversely, headache sufferers receiving a cognitive treatment, with no biofeedback, reported a significant reduction in headache although there was no EMG reduction in this group. As Turk et al. (80) indicate, it appears that some individuals with very high levels of frontalis EMG report few or no tension headaches, while others with relatively low EMG levels report frequent headaches. All these data raise doubts about the relationship between muscle tension and pain. At the same time, some investigations have shown a positive relationship between EMG and clinical pain (13, 37). See Budzynski (11), Philips (63), and Turk et al. (80) for a more complete discussion of this important issue.

Unless it can be demonstrated that EMG feedback results in EMG reduction, which in turn is associated with headache reduction, basic questions arise about whether the biofeedback treatment effects are attributable to the biofeedback per se or to "nonspecific" treatment effects. In reviewing this issue, Turk et al. (80, p. 1326) come to the conclusion that "the evidence does not convincingly demonstrate that frontalis EMG reduction and self-report of tension headaches are concordant. Thus it seems premature to conclude that the positive effects of biofeedback approaches, when indeed they occur, are a function of increasingly voluntary control of frontalis muscle activity." In a similar vein, Beaty and Haynes (6) concluded that the contribution of nonspecific placebo, expectancy and demand factors have not been adequately controlled.*

A second fundamental question which has been raised concerns the cost-effectiveness of frontalis EMG feedback for the treatment of tension headache. This issue has been reviewed recently by Budzynski (11), Jessup et al. (43), Silver and Blanchard (71) and Turk et al. (80). Jessup et al. (43, p. 240) concluded that "in controlled studies, simply teaching headache sufferers to relax was consistently as effective as EMG biofeedback and superior to control conditions." They base this conclusion on studies such as that conducted by Chesney and Shelton (17). These investigators compared four experimental conditions, namely, relaxation training, EMG feedback, combined relaxation and feedback, and no treatment control. Jessup et al. (43) calculated that, in Chesney and Shelton's study, headache frequency decreased 75% with relaxation, 42% with feedback, 77% with the combined treatment and 12% among controls. Headache duration decreased 53% with relaxation, *increased* 19% with feedback, decreased 77% with combined treatment and decreased 1% among controls. Changes in intensity were as follows: relaxation, 47% reduction; feedback, 38% decrease; combined, 68% decrease; control, 20% increase. Chesney and Shelton (17) found that while the relaxation and combined treatment resulted in significant improvement relative to untreated controls, biofeedback alone did not. Both the relaxation and combined treatments resulted in significantly more reduction in headache duration than did biofeedback alone. Similarly, Gray et al. (35) recently found relaxation training to be more effective than EMG feedback in the treatment of tension headache immediately after treatment, although at follow-up (1–6 months after treatment) no differences were observed across treatment groups. Two studies (18, 37) have found relaxation training and EMG feedback equally effective in reducing tension headache.

---

* F. Andrasik and K. A. Holroyd published an important paper related to this issue (A test of specific and nonspecific effects in the biofeedback treatment of tension headache. *Journal of Consulting and Clinical Psychology*, 1980, *48:* 575–586) after the present chapter had been written. These investigators found that subjects trained to produce either increased, stable, or decreased frontalis EMG levels all showed significant improvement in headache compared with a no treatment control group. No differences in improvement were found across the three biofeedback treatment conditions. This pattern of results suggests that learned EMG changes did not play a major role in the improved clinical reports.

The studies just reviewed suggest that relaxation training is at least as effective as EMG feedback for treating tension headache. One study, Hutchings and Reinking (40), which was quite similar to that of Chesney and Shelton (17), found EMG feedback and combined relaxation-feedback to be superior to relaxation training alone. This appears to be the only study showing EMG feedback to be superior to relaxation training. However, in a subsequent report, Reinking (described by Silver and Blanchard (71)) found that the combined treatment was superior to the other two treatments at the end of treatment and at a 3-month follow-up. But at 6- and 12-month follow-ups, there was no evidence of significant differences across treatment conditions; less than 50% of Ss available for these follow-ups were reporting success. At follow-up, Reinking found that significantly more "success" than "failure" patients reported that they were continuing to practice. Budzynski et al. (13) have also stressed the importance of daily home practice as a supplement to EMG biofeedback training. While a number of controlled studies of EMG feedback have shown treatment benefits over brief follow-up periods of 4 months or less (43), Reinking's follow-up data suggest there is a need for more long-term follow-up information.

As they have weighed the evidence, most recent reviewers have concluded that there are no empirical grounds for believing that frontalis EMG biofeedback is more effective than relaxation training, which is much more cost-efficient (43, 71, 80). While Belar (8) agrees with this conclusion, she has argued that we should not consider the question settled. She notes, for instance, that the studies on which the conclusion is based have relied primarily on undergraduates with headache problems who may not be representative of the clinical population at large. She also suggests that procedural refinements may yield more impressive results from biofeedback treatment.

Biofeedback procedures have been used to treat migraine as well as muscle contraction headaches. The best known biofeedback treatment for migraine headache involves training patients to raise their hand temperature. This strategy was suggested by a serendipitous finding: a subject participating in an experiment at the Menninger Foundation noted that while she was experiencing an increase in hand temperature, she aborted a migraine headache (68). This prompted Sargent et al. (67, 69) to explore the effectiveness of a migraine treatment program in which patients were taught to raise hand temperature relative to forehead temperature using a combination of thermal feedback and autogenic training (which involved using visual, auditory and somatic imagery to promote the physiological change). Although the etiology of migraine headache is not clearly understood, it does appear to be associated with excessive cranial-vascular responsivity (3). In developing the rationale for their treatment, Sargent et al. (69) suggested that the vascular dysfunction was stress related and was triggered by activation of the sympathetic nervous system. They viewed hand warming training as a potentially effective treatment on the assumption that the therapy taught patients to "'turn off' excessive sympathetic outflow" (69, p. 419).

Data from early uncontrolled treatment studies were encouraging. For instance, Sargent et al. (69) treated 42 migraine sufferers using the combination of biofeedback and autogenic training. Treatment was self-administered at home. Initially, portable equipment was used for training until the S had mastered hand warming. At this point, hand warming was practiced without the machine on alternate days. Then the machine was withdrawn completely (usually within a month of the beginning of training), and the S was expected to continue to practice daily without feedback. Eighty-one percent of the patients were deemed improved (8/42 no improvement, 18/42 slight to moderate improvement, 16/42 good to very good improvement). Since there is no control for regression effects, expectancy or other variables which could account for changes in self-reported headache activity, evidence from such uncontrolled studies is not conclusive.

Subsequent controlled studies have raised questions about the efficacy of the treatment. Jessup et al. (43) indicate that the results of controlled studies have, on balance, been discouraging. Their assessment is based on recent studies, most of which have not yet been published except in abstract form. Beasley (5) reported that a combination of autogenic training, relaxation exercises and temperature feedback (although not temperature feedback alone) resulted in significant improvement relative to an untreated control group. However, Jessup (42) found no differences between autogenic-temperature feedback training and untreated controls. Kewman (45) also found that hand warming feedback training did not result in significant improvement relative to untreated controls. While Blanchard et al. (10) found autogenic-temperature feedback training effective relative to an untreated control group on some measures, progressive relaxation training was as effective as the more elaborate intervention. Based on these findings, it would seem premature to conclude that temperature feedback (even with autogenic training) can be considered a cost-effective treatment of proven value. While this conclusion appears to be consistent with that of most recent reviewers (43, 71, 80), Diamond et al. (20) are somewhat more positive. The latter conclude that "biofeedback has proven to be a worthwhile therapeutic modality in the treatment of vascular headaches, but many factors have yet to be explored" (p. 404). Their more optimistic conclusion seems to be based largely on data from uncontrolled studies in which biofeedback was often used in conjunction with other modalities. Despite the optimism of Diamond et al. (20), a more cautious conclusion seems to be in order if more credence is placed in controlled studies (although, again it should be emphasized that many of the controlled studies have not been published in full and, therefore, have not yet been widely scrutinized).

The credibility of temperature training has been called into question by studies which raise doubts about the relationship between hand warming and changes in pain reports (43, 80). Kewman (45) reported that individual Ss who learned to raise finger temperature did not experience more symptomatic relief than Ss who failed to learn to raise their temperature. Moreover, Kewman (45) and Jessup (42) both found that hand cooling, hand warming and no treatment resulted in comparable amounts of clinical improvement. The observation that training in hand cooling resulted in as much improvement as training in hand warming and that neither of these treatments outperformed untreated controls raises serious questions about whether the positive results obtained in the less well-controlled studies were due to temperature change training per se or to nonspecific treatment effects. Kewman (45, p. 3400B) concluded from his data that "regression to the mean and placebo factors appear to contribute substantially to the treatment effect." It might be noted that Turin and Johnson (77) found that finger warming training did lead to headache relief while finger cooling training did not: hence, the data on this issue are not entirely clear-cut.

Another form of biofeedback—cephalic blood volume pulse (BVP) feedback—has been used to treat migraine (9, 21, 22, 32, 73). This form of treatment is intended to reduce migraine by providing direct training in the constriction of cephalic arteries. Friar and Beatty (32) found that BVP feedback significantly reduced migraine, while a control treatment (finger vasoconstriction training) did not. Bild and Adams (9) reported more improvement in response to BVP feedback than to EMG feedback or no treatment. While these controlled studies are encouraging, further research is required before final conclusions can be drawn about the value of this treatment. Bild and Adams (9), for instance, did not find consistent, statistically significant evidence of the superiority of BVP feedback across all measures (perhaps because there were only 19 Ss distributed across the three treatment conditions). Also, follow-ups have either been brief (9) or nonexistent (32) in the controlled studies.

It might be noted in passing that biofeedback has been used to treat pain syndromes other than muscle contraction and migraine headache. Jessup et al. (43) and Turk et al. (80) have cited quite a large number of studies which have described the use of various forms of biofeedback in problems which include low back pain, menstrual distress, neck pain, peptic ulcer, pyelonephritis, posttraumatic head pain, Raynaud's disease, rheumatoid arthritis, temporomandibular joint pain and writer's cramp. Most of these reports are uncontrolled case descriptions.

Biofeedback seems to be in wide use. A review of the literature raises serious questions about the empirical justification for the current enthusiasm. While some applications are promising, more evidence is required about their mode of action and efficacy (in absolute terms or relative to less complex and expensive treatment alternatives) before they can be promoted as the unequivocal treatment of choice. One comes away from this literature with a sense that relaxation training is a simple, cost-effective intervention which may be quite useful in the treatment of headache.

Meichenbaum (54) has suggested that biofeedback therapists have been rather mechanical and narrowly focused in their approach to therapy. He suggests that biofeedback treatments should be incorporated into a more comprehensive self-control treatment regimen and offers some suggestions for doing this. Meichenbaum's views seem to accord with those of Mitchell and White (62), who have noted that biofeedback treatments for (headache) pain tend to focus intervention on the last link in the behavioral chain that precedes pain. Situational and psychological antecedents which may elicit the presumed physiological change tend to be ignored. Mitchell and White argue that more comprehensive skill training for coping with environmental stress should be included to maximize therapeutic benefit. They have developed a comprehensive skill training program which is reviewed below.

COGNITIVE BEHAVIORAL SKILL TRAINING

Recently, there has been a growing tendency to construe clinical problems in terms of skill deficits in either the cognitive or behavioral domains. From this point of view, the goal of therapy is to assist the client to develop adaptive cognitive and behavioral skills. Mahoney and Arnkoff (50) and Meichenbaum (55) recently have reviewed such interventions. Although the general approach is relatively new, a number of investigators have explored its utility in the treatment of pain. Much of this work has focused on acute pain induced in undergraduates in a laboratory situation. While this work is exciting, it will not be reviewed here: a recent, detailed review is available (78). Nor will application of cognitive interventions to acute pain situations (e.g., surgery) be considered (see Turk and Genest (79), for a recent review). The focus will be limited to studies conducted with clinical populations presenting with recurrent or chronic pain problems.

A comprehensive cognitive-behavioral approach to treating migraine headache has been described by Mitchell and his colleagues (59–62). Mitchell's treatment includes relaxation training, systematic desensitization, assertiveness training, and training in problem solving for day-to-day living. In a series of controlled studies, Mitchell has demonstrated that this treatment is more effective than no treatment (59). Moreover, the comprehensive treatment program has been found to be more effective than relaxation alone, systematic desensitization alone, or monitoring of headache alone (60). The effects of the treatment have been impressive. For instance, the combined treatment resulted in a 95% mean reduction in headache frequency and an 80% mean reduction in headache duration (vs. mean reductions of 7% and 9%, respectively, among untreated controls). The combined treatment was limited to 15 sessions, 50–60 min each, two sessions per week (60).

Mitchell and White (62) conducted a sequential treatment study in which they evaluated the efficacy of different components of a comprehensive behavioral self-management program. The general objective of the complete program is to teach "people to analyze and identify problems in their own personal environments and behaviors (both overt and covert), to work out their own management strategies, and to self-apply control techniques aimed at modifying both their environment and their reactions to that environment" (p. 214). The components of the complete program include 1) self-recording (of the frequency of headaches), 2) self-monitoring (self-observing and recording antecedent stress cues), 3) training in three core self-control skills—physical and mental relaxation and self-desensitization (skill acquisition stage 1), and 4) training in 13 further self-control skills—including rational thinking, projected rehearsal and imaginal modeling (skill acquisition stage 2).

Twelve migraine patients were treated. Participants had had headaches for 4 to 13 years (average, 7.1). Pretreatment frequency of migraines ranged from 9 to 17 (mean, 13.6) per 4-week period. Subjects were randomly assigned to one of four conditions: self-recording (SR), self-monitoring (SM), self-monitoring and skill acquisition stage 1 (SMS_1) and self-monitoring and skill acquisition stages 1 and 2 ($SMS_{1,2}$). Subjects were seen on a group basis, with all 12 receiving the first component (SR), after which SR Ss dropped out and the remaining 9 received SM. In a similar fashion, 3 Ss dropped out after each stage of treatment, so that only 3 Ss received the full program. Each stage lasted 12 weeks, although therapeutic contact was minimal: there was only one contact per phase. The two skill acquisition interventions were conducted via 30-min introductory prerecorded audio tapes; Ss were then given additional skill-training audio tapes to take home with them.

Mean headache frequency remained virtually unchanged among all Ss during the first two phases. At the end of 1 year from the beginning of the treatment, Ss who received only SR or SR and SM still showed virtually no change in headache frequency. These results indicated that self-recording and self-monitoring were not sufficient to reduce headaches. However, each of the skill acquisition treatments resulted in a decrease in headache. Hence, at the end of treatment, Ss who received the complete package were reporting significantly fewer headaches (mean = 3.7 per month) than Ss who received only the first stage of skill acquisition (mean = 6.4 per month). Both of these skill acquisition groups had fewer headaches than SR (mean = 13.2 per month) and SM (mean = 12.7 per month) Ss. At a follow-up 3 months later, SMS_1 Ss reported an average of 6.2 headaches per month and $SMS_{1,2}$ Ss reported 2.3 per month. These results are especially remarkable when it is recalled that therapist contact was minimal, with therapy essentially conducted by audio-tape.

It might be noted that the study relied upon self-report data for the evaluation of treatment effectiveness. Such data is susceptible to subject response bias and demand characteristics. Subjects who saw themselves receiving more treatment as their fellow group participants dropped out of the study could clearly infer that they were receiving more intensive treatment. It could be argued that this could have created demand characteristics that might lead them to report increased improvement in response to the successive skill training stages. Assuming that the findings can be confirmed using a design which rules out this problem, this appears to be a promising approach to treatment which is both effective and cost-efficient.

A second approach to skill training therapy has been described by Holroyd and his colleagues. These investigators have worked with tension headache patients. In an initial study (39), three experimental conditions were compared: stress-coping training, EMG feedback assisted relaxation training, and waiting-list control. Treatment was conducted on an individual basis during eight biweekly 45-min sessions. Stress-coping training procedures were based on the work of Beck (7), Goldfried et al. (33) and Meichenbaum (55). The treatment rationale presented to the subject was that disturbing moods and behaviors resulted from certain thought processes or cognitions. Tension headache was put into this category of a stress-response determined by thoughts about a situation; specific examples illustrated a variety of events that might be seen as stressful by different persons and the way in which cognitions were responsible for stress and headache. In this way the clients were induced to attribute their headaches to specific maladaptive cognitions; the provision of this sort of rationale may be of therapeutic value in and of itself (81). After describing the rationale for treatment, the client and therapist identified 1) the cues that trigger tension, 2) the client's typical response to tension, 3) the client's thoughts prior to, during and after awareness of tension, and 4) the ways in which cognitions appeared to contribute to the client's tension and headache. This sort of exercise was intended to teach the client to identify his own cognitive components of distress and provide him with evidence for a cognitive interpretation of his problem. It was suspected that self-monitoring of cognitions would itself influence subsequent responses (44). Thought patterns producing distress were attributed to unrealistic beliefs which have to be identified and altered. As clients became conversant with the above tasks, they learned to interrupt the behavioral sequence leading to their distress by using signs of impending distress as signals to employ stress-reducing cognitive strategies including "cognitive reappraisal," "attention deployment" and "fantasy or imagery" (48). After the third training session the clients were encouraged to apply this skill package at the first sign of headache.

The results showed that only the cognitive coping skills training proved effective. This group showed significant improvement in headache relative to both the biofeedback and untreated controls at both the posttreatment and the follow-up assessments. The latter two groups did not differ significantly in headache at either the posttreatment or the follow-up assessment. Changes in headache activity were quite impressive among skill training participants. Although only adjusted means are presented for the post-test and follow-up, it appears that average weekly headache duration dropped from 20.6 hours to less than half that amount at post-test and follow-up among coping skills participants. Untreated controls remained virtually unchanged. These data, along with changes in other headache parameters, indicate the treatment was significant clinically as well as statistically. All treatment Ss who had been regularly using medication reported decreases in medication use. Moreover, the coping skills (and the biofeedback) group reported fewer general psychosomatic complaints than did controls at the end of treatment. This suggests that the coping skills training, which is not tailored specifically to headaches, may prove effective in treating other psychosomatic disorders as well.

A second study (38) suggested that this sort of skill training could be conducted both effectively and economically using group treatment. Participants were tension headache sufferers who responded to a newspaper announcement of the treatment program. There were four treatment conditions: cognitive self-control (directed at modifying stress-related maladaptive cognitions), combined cognitive self-control and relaxation training, headache discussion (the focus was on discussing the historical roots of symptoms rather than on the development of coping skills), and an untreated control group. Treatment of the first three conditions was conducted on a group basis in five weekly 1¾-hr sessions. Both of the self-control groups and the headache discussion group showed significant reduction in headache relative to the untreated controls: the improvement was maintained at a 6 week follow-up.

The study confirmed that stress management skill training can produce significant symptomatic improvement. However, the fact that the headache discussion group showed a comparable level of improvement raises questions about the active ingredients of the skill training interventions. When Holroyd and Andrasik (38) interviewed participants following treatment, they discovered that all but one of the members of the headache discussion group had spontaneously devised apparently effective cognitive coping measures, enabling the users to reevaluate their stressors as less worrisome. In fact, the only participant who did not report devising such cognitive self-control measures also showed the least improvement in headache activity. On the basis of these retrospective interviews, Holroyd and Andrasik suggest that the improvement reported by the headache discussion group may have resulted from members of this treatment group developing cognitive coping strategies on their own. If this interpretation is accurate, it implies that a substantial proportion of clinical patients have an affinity for using cognitive coping strategies. This would suggest that this approach to treatment might be highly productive. Alternatively, the finding of no difference between the general discussion and skill training groups may imply that the apparent efficacy of the skill training was due to nonspecific effects such as demand characteristics. At the same time, it should be remembered that training was superior to biofeedback in the study by Holroyd et al. (39), even though biofeedback was rated as a highly credible treatment by Ss who received it: this result suggests that in that study, at least, the efficacy of skill training cannot easily be discounted by attributing it to nonspecific effects.

Bakal et al. (4) recently evaluated a cognitive behavioral treatment with a mixed group of headache sufferers. The sample included persons diagnosed as having muscle contraction, migraine, or combined muscle contraction-migraine headaches based on a neurological examination. It is noteworthy that the patients were referred for treatment by family practitioners and neurologists. The mean duration of the headache problem was 16.8 years, and the headaches were difficult to control with medication. Hence, it appears that this was a bonafide clinical sample.

The treatment procedure followed Meichenbaum's (55) model of self-control training which construes treatment as a three-stage process. Meichenbaum has suggested treatment be viewed as consisting of an observational phase (the objective is for the client and therapist alike to collect and examine data pertinent to the presenting problem), an educational phase (during which a conceptual framework is developed for understanding the problem), and a skill acquisition phase (during which the patient learns to modify his behavior).

During the observational phase, Bakal et al. (4) asked patients to chart headache activity on a form which permitted easy recording of fairly detailed information. The 3-week self-observation period was intended not only to provide baseline data but also to have patients observe the thoughts, feelings and sensations that preceded and accompanied headaches. Cognitive behavioral therapists tend to view the client as an active collaborator in the treatment process; Bakal et al. (4) note that the self-observation procedure lays the groundwork for developing this sort of therapeutic relationship.

This self-observation period was followed by 12 weekly treatment sessions, conducted on an individual basis. The first objective during these sessions (educational phase) was to encourage patients to acquire a more fine-grained understanding of their problem, an understanding which would permit them to view previously undifferentiated attacks as consisting of a number of identifiable, smaller components. The therapist presented a psychophysiological model of headache which emphasized the interplay between presumed physiological mechanisms underlying headache activity (e.g., heightened muscle tension) and psychological processes (sensations and cognitions) which precede and accompany headache attacks. During these early sessions with the therapist, relaxation training and five sessions of EMG biofeedback training were provided. Both forms of training were introduced primarily to encourage patients to observe changes in sensations, thoughts, and feelings which were associated with relaxation.

The final (skill acquisition) phase occurred during sessions 8–12. Patients were trained to use attention focusing, imagery production, and thought management as described by Turk (78). In general, these cognitive skills are intended to reduce psychological reaction to pain by training the client to mentally create and focus on pleasant physical sensations, substitute rational coping self-statements for catastrophic thoughts, etc. Turk (78) has outlined a rich array of such strategies. During these sessions, Bakal et al. (4) promoted transfer of the acquired skills to the patient's natural environment through homework assignments intended to foster consolidation and generalization of the newly acquired skills.

Posttreatment and follow-up data were collected by self-monitoring over a 14-day period immediately following treatment and for an additional 14 days 6 months after the end of treatment. Significant improvement was found on all measures. Mean daily headache hours dropped from 9.1 (pre) to 4.9 (post) and was 3.7 at follow-up. A "daily headache index" measure (hours of headache × intensity at each hour ÷ number of days in observation period) showed a decrease from 19.4 at pretest to 10.4 at posttest and 8.2 at follow-up. Average number of pills taken per day dropped from 1.7 at pretest to 0.8 at posttest and 0.5 at follow-up. These decreases appear to be clinically meaningful as well as statistically significant.

Treatment outcome was quite variable across subjects. Interestingly, positive outcome was not associated with clinical diagnosis (muscle contraction, migraine, and combined patients responded equally well) nor was outcome associated with sex, age, years of reported headache, location of pain, time of onset (during the day), or symptoms which accompanied headache. However, it was found that patients who experienced continuous or near-continuous pain during the waking hours tended to realize little benefit from the treatment. Patients who had reported less than 8 hr of head pain per day showed a 52% reduction in daily headache hours; those who had reported 8–14.9 hr of headache per day had a 61% reduction in headache hours; but those who had reported 15 or more waking hours of pain dropped a mere 11% in number of headache hours.

The results of this study appear encouraging especially in light of the fact that most patients had chronic problems that had not responded well to traditional medical treatments. However, it is important to note that no control group was included. Also, at the time the report was written, only 20 of the 45 subjects had completed the 6 month follow-up. Although further data are required to assess the efficacy of this type of cognitive behavioral intervention, the preliminary data from this impressive clinical trial suggest that such treatment may be useful in the management of even severe, chronic problems.

A number of other recent papers have described cognitive or cognitive-behavioral approaches to the treatment of chronic pain. For example, Levendusky and Pankratz (49) reported a case study in which a man experiencing abdominal pain was treated using a program of relaxation, covert imagery, and cognitive relabeling. Cautela (16) has described procedures designed to modify pain responses by means of covert conditioning. Rybstein-Blinchik (65) recently has published a controlled study which suggests that chronic pain patients may benefit from therapy designed to induce a cognitive reinterpretation and relabeling of pain related experience.

Cognitive coping strategies have been found effective in modifying acute pain induced in laboratory situations. While many of these strategies have not yet been evaluated with chronic pain patients, they may have clinical value. Reviews of such strategies are available in Meichenbaum (55), Meichenbaum and Turk (57) and Turk (78). A book now in preparation by Turk, Meichenbaum and Genest is likely to be a valuable contribution to the literature on cognitive behavioral strategies for treating pain.

Summary and Integration

Behavioral approaches to the treatment of common pain problems are being utilized increasingly. Operant programs have demonstrated what appear to be impressive results with long-term chronic pain patients who have not responded well to other treatments. However, the available data are difficult to interpret with confidence because of a lack of controlled research and high attrition rates at follow-up. The absence of control groups is of particular concern since it has been reported that up to 50% of low back pain patients may report relief with no surgery and conservative management (23). While biofeedback seems to be in wide use, recent reviews (43, 71, 80) suggest that the current enthusiasm for this approach does not have a compelling empirical basis. There is some question about 1) the efficacy of common biofeedback treatments, especially in relation to less expensive alternatives, and 2) the extent to which clinical improvement is mediated by specific treatment effects. At the same time, relaxation training does appear to have therapeutic value and to be cost-effective. Cognitive behavioral skill training approaches appear to hold promise; however, their potential value and limitations cannot be defined conclusively without further evaluation. If there is some uncertainty about the efficacy of behavioral treatment interventions, this is not surprising given that behaviorally oriented clinical researchers have only recently become interested in the treatment of chronic pain. It is startling to realize that the oldest intervention study cited in this review was published in 1968. Except for individual pioneering efforts in each of the three areas, most of the research has been published within the past 5 years.

As the field develops, both research and clinical work will benefit from construction of integrative models which specify psychological variables that influence the pain experience and the patterns of interplay among these variables. At present, operant, psychophysiological, and cognitive-behavioral conceptualizations remain relatively unintegrated, although each perspective is clearly important in its own right. A complete understanding of the psychological aspects of the pain experience (or of any individual pain patient's problem) requires that all these perspectives be considered. Further basic research is required before we have available a model for making rational, systematic, data-based decisions about the clinical management of individual pain patients. As noted above, for instance, there is still considerable debate about what role, if any, muscle contraction plays in "muscle contraction" headache. Also, although there is a belief that maladaptive cognitions may contribute significantly to some patients' problems, there is not yet a well-established set of clinical procedures for assessing cognition (56). Compelling guidelines for clinical decision making (which take into account environmental, psychophysiological, cognitive, and behavioral variables) are likely to emerge only as such issues are clarified. Even now, however, the clinician has available a diverse set of procedures which seem to hold promise, although final data are not in.

There is some evidence that treatment may be more effective when interventions are targeted at more than one of the psychological systems (environmental, psychophysiological, cognitive, behavioral) that potentially influence the pain experience. For instance, Reeves (64) described a systematic case study in which a tension headache patient was taught to use coping self-statements in stressful situations. The patient also learned to monitor cognitions and to substitute positive for negative thoughts. This cognitive intervention resulted in a 33% reduction in headaches. Next, 6 weeks of frontalis EMG feedback was provided. This resulted in a further 33% reduction in headaches. While this is an uncontrolled (although systematic) case study and data cannot be interpreted with complete confidence, it does suggest that clinical results may be enhanced if interventions are comprehensive. Other reports of integrative approaches have been described recently (34, 46, 47). A catholic approach which blends environmental, psychophysiological, cognitive, and behavioral interventions in a rational manner tailored to the specific problems of individual patients appears to be called for.

REFERENCES

1. AMERICAN MEDICAL ASSOCIATION. Report of the Ad Hoc Committee on the classification of headache. J. A. M. A. 179: 717–718, 1962.
2. ANDERSON, T. P., COLE, T. M., GULLICKSON, G., HUDGENS, A., AND ROBERTS, A. H. Behavior modification of chronic pain. Clin. Orthop., 129: 96–100, 1977.
3. BAKAL, D. H. Headache: A biopsychological perspective. Psychol. Bull., 82: 369–382, 1975.
4. BAKAL, D. A., DEMJEN, S., AND KAGANOV, J. A. Cognitive Behavioral Treatment of Headache. Unpublished manuscript. University of Calgary, 1980.
5. BEASLEY, J. Biofeedback in the treatment of migraine headaches. Dissert. Abstr. Intern., 36: 5850B–5851B, 1976.

6. BEATY, E. T., AND HAYNES, S. N. Behavioral intervention with muscle-contraction headache: A review. *Psychosom. Med.*, *41:* 165–180, 1979.
7. BECK, A. T. *Cognitive Therapy and the Emotional Disorders.* International Universities Press, New York, 1976.
8. BELAR, C. D. A comment on Silver and Blanchard's (1978) review of the treatment of tension headaches via EMG feedback and relaxation training. *J. Behav. Med.*, *2:* 215–220, 1979.
9. BILD, R., AND ADAMS, H. E. Modification of migraine headaches by cephalic blood volume pulse and EMG biofeedback. *J. Consult. Clin. Psychol.*, *48:* 51–57, 1980.
10. BLANCHARD, E., THEOBALD, D., WILLIAMSON, D., SILVER, B., AND BROWN, D. Temperature biofeedback in the treatment of migraine headaches. *Arch. Gen. Psychiatry*, *35:* 581–588, 1978.
11. BUDZYNSKI, T. Biofeedback in the treatment of muscle contraction (tension) headache. *Biofeedback Self Regul.*, *3:* 409–434, 1978.
12. BUDZYNSKI, T. H., STOYVA, J. M., AND ADLER, C. S. Feedback-induced muscle relaxation: Application to tension headache. *J. Behav. Ther. Exp. Psychiatry*, *1:* 205–211, 1970.
13. BUDZYNSKI, T. H., STOYVA, J. M., ADLER, C. S., AND MULLANEY, D. J. EMG biofeedback and tension headache: A controlled outcome study. *Psychosom. Med.*, *35:* 484–496, 1973.
14. CAIRNS, D., AND PASINO, J. A. Comparison of verbal reinforcement and feedback in operant treatment of disability due to low back pain. *Behav. Ther.*, *8:* 621–630, 1977.
15. CAIRNS, D., THOMAS, L., MOONEY, V., AND PACE, J. B. A comprehensive treatment approach to low back pain. *Pain*, *2:* 301–308, 1976.
16. CAUTELA, J. R. The use of covert conditioning in modifying pain behavior. *J. Behav. Ther. Exp. Psychiatry*, *8:* 45–52, 1977.
17. CHESNEY, M., AND SHELTON, J. L. A comparison of muscle relaxation and electromyogram biofeedback treatments for muscle contraction headache. *J. Behav. Ther. Exp. Psychiatry*, *7:* 221–225, 1976.
18. COX, D. J., FREUNDLICH, A., AND MEYER, R. G. Differential effectiveness of electromyograph feedback, verbal relaxation instructions, and medication placebo with tension headaches. *J. Consult. Clin. Psychology*, *43:* 892–899, 1975.
19. DALESSIO, D. J. *Wolff's Headache and Other Head Pain.* Oxford University Press, New York, 1972.
20. DIAMOND, S., DIAMOND-FALK, J., AND DEVENO, T. Biofeedback in the treatment of vascular headache. *Biofeedback Self Regul.*, *3:* 385–408, 1978.
21. FEUERSTEIN, M., AND ADAMS, H. E. Cephalic vasomotor feedback in the modification of migraine headaches. *Biofeedback Self Regul.*, *2:* 241–253, 1977.
22. FEUERSTEIN, M., ADAMS, H. E., AND BEIMAN, I. Cephalic vasomotor and electromyographic feedback in the treatment of combined muscle contraction and migraine headaches in a geriatric case. *Headache*, *16:* 232–253, 1976.
23. FINNESON, B. E. *Low Back Pain.* Lippincott, Philadelphia, 1973.
24. FINNESON, B. E. Modulating effect of secondary gain on the low back pain syndrome. In *Advances in Pain Research and Therapy*, Vol. 1, edited by J. J. Bonica and D. Albe-Fessard. Raven, New York, 1976.
25. FORDYCE, W. E. Treating chronic pain by contingency management. In *Advances in Neurology*, Vol. 4, edited by J. J. Bonica. Raven Press, New York, 1974.
26. FORDYCE, W. E. Pain viewed as learned behavior. In *Advances in Neurology*, Vol. 4, edited by J. J. Bonica. Raven Press, New York, 1974.
27. FORDYCE, W. E. *Behavioral Methods for Chronic Pain and Illness.* C. V. Mosby, St. Louis, 1976.
28. FORDYCE, W. E. Environmental factors in the genesis of low back pain. In *Advances in Pain Research and Therapy*, Vol. 3, edited by J. J. Bonica, J. C. Liebeskind, and D. G. Albe-Fessard. Raven Press, New York, 1979.

29. FORDYCE, W. E., FOWLER, R. S., AND DeLATEUR, B. An application of behavior modification technique to a problem of chronic pain. *Behav. Res. Ther.*, 6: 105–107, 1968.
30. FORDYCE, W. E., FOWLER, R. S., LEHMANN, J. F., DeLATEUR, B. J., SAND, P. L., AND TRIESCHMAN, R. B. Operant conditioning in the treatment of chronic pain. *Arch. Phys. Med. Rehabil.*, 54: 399–408, 1973.
31. FOWLER, R. S., FORDYCE, W. E., AND BERNI, R. Operant conditioning in chronic illness. *Am. J. Nurs.*, 69: 1226–1228, 1969.
32. FRIAR, L. R., AND BEATTY, J. Migraine: Management by trained control of vasoconstriction. *J. Consult. Clin. Psychol.*, 44: 46–53, 1976.
33. GOLDFRIED, M. R., DECENTECCO, E. T., AND WEINBERG, L. Systematic rational restructuring as a self-control technique. *Behav. Ther.*, 5: 247–254, 1974.
34. GOTTLIEB, H., STRITE, L. C., KOLLER, R., MADORSKY, A., HOCKERSMITH, V., KLEEMAN, M., AND WAGNER, J. Comprehensive rehabilitation of patients having chronic low back pain. *Arch. Phys. Med. Rehabil.*, 58: 101–108, 1977.
35. GRAY, C. L., LYLE, R. C., McGUIRE, R. J., AND PECK, D. F. Electrode placement, EMG feedback, and relaxation for tension headaches. *Behav. Res. Ther.*, 18: 19–23, 1980.
36. GREENHOOT, J. H., AND STERNBACH, R. A. Conjoint treatment of chronic pain. In *Advances in Neurology*, Vol. 4, edited by J. J. Bonica. Raven Press, New York, 1974.
37. HAYNES, S. N., GRIFFIN, P., MOONEY, D., AND PARISE, M. Electromyographic biofeedback and relaxation instructions in the treatment of muscle contraction headaches. *Behav. Ther.*, 6: 672–678, 1975.
38. HOLROYD, K. A., AND ANDRASIK, F. Coping and the self-control of chronic tension headache. *J. Consult. Clin. Psychol.*, 46: 1036–1045, 1978.
39. HOLROYD, K. A., ANDRASIK, F., AND WESTBROOK, T. Cognitive control of tension headache. *Cognit. Ther. Res.*, 1: 121–133, 1977.
40. HUTCHINGS, D. F., AND REINKING, R. H. Tension headaches: What form of therapy is most effective? *Biofeedback Self Regul.*, 1: 183–190, 1976.
41. IGNELZI, R. J., STERNBACH, R. A., AND TIMMERMANS, G. The pain ward follow-up analyses. *Pain*, 3: 277–280, 1977.
42. JESSUP, B. A. Autogenic biofeedback training for migraine: A bidirectional control group study. Unpublished manuscript. Described in Jessup et al. (43).
43. JESSUP, B. A., NEUFELD, W. J., AND MERSKEY, H. Biofeedback therapy for headache and other pain: An evaluative review. *Pain*, 7: 225–270, 1979.
44. KANFER, F. H. The maintenance of behavior by self-generated stimuli and reinforcement. In *The Psychology of Private Events*, edited by A. Jacobs and L. B. Sachs. Academic Press, New York, 1971.
45. KEWMAN, D. G. Voluntary control of digital skin temperature for treatment of migraine headaches. *Dissert. Abstr. Intern.*, 38: 3399B–3400B, 1978.
46. KHATAMI, M., AND RUSH, A. J. A pilot study of the treatment of outpatients with chronic pain: Symptom control, stimulus control, and social system intervention. *Pain*, 5: 163–172, 1979.
47. KHATAMI, M., WOODY, G., AND O'BRIEN, C. Chronic pain and narcotic addiction: A multitherapeutic approach—a pilot study. *Compr. Psychiatry*, 25: 55–60, 1979.
48. LAZARUS, R., AVERILL, J., AND OPTON, E. The psychology of coping: Issues of research and assessment. In *Coping and Adaptation*, edited by G. Coelho, D. Hamburg, and J. Adams. Basic Books, New York, 1974.
49. LEVENDUSKY, P., AND PANKRATZ, L. Self-control techniques as an alternative to pain medication. *J. Abnorm. Psychol.*, 84: 165–168, 1975.
50. MAHONEY, M. J., AND ARNKOFF, D. Cognitive and self-control therapies. In *Handbook of Psychotherapy and Behavior Change*, Ed. 2, edited by S. L. Garfield and A. E. Bergin. Wiley, New York, 1978.
51. MARTIN, M. J. Tension headache: A psychiatric study. *Headache*, 6: 47–54, 1966.

52. MARTIN, M. J. Muscle-contraction headache. *Psychosomatics, 13:* 16–19, 1972.
53. MARUTA, T., SWANSON, D. W., AND SWENSON, W. M. Chronic pain: Which patients may a pain management program help? *Pain, 7:* 321–329, 1979.
54. MEICHENBAUM, D. Cognitive factors in biofeedback therapy. *Biofeedback Self Regul., 1:* 201–216, 1976.
55. MEICHENBAUM, D. *Cognitive-Behavior Modification: An Integrative Approach.* New York. Plenum Press, 1977.
56. MEICHENBAUM, D., AND CAMERON, R. Issues in cognitive assessment: An overview. In *Cognitive Assessment.* edited by T. Merluzzi, C. Glass, and M. Genest. Guilford Press, New York, in press.
57. MEICHENBAUM, D., AND TURK, D. C. The cognitive behavioral management of anxiety, anger and pain. In *The Behavioral Management of Anxiety, Depression and Pain.* edited by P. Davidson. Bruner Mazel, New York, 1976.
58. MILLER, N. E. Biofeedback and visceral learning. *Annu. Rev. Psychol., 29:* 373–404, 1978.
59. MITCHELL, K. R. Note on treatment of migraine using behavior therapy techniques. *Psychol. Rep., 28:* 171–172, 1971.
60. MITCHELL, K. R., AND MITCHELL, D. M. Migraine: An exploratory treatment application of programmed behavior therapy techniques. *J. Psychosom. Res., 15:* 137–157, 1971.
61. MITCHELL, K. R., AND WHITE, R. G. Control of migraine headache by behavioral self-management: A controlled case study. *Headache, 16:* 178–184, 1976.
62. MITCHELL, K. R., AND WHITE, R. G. Behavioral self-management: An application to the problem of migraine headaches. *Behav. Ther., 8:* 213–222, 1977.
63. PHILIPS, C. Tension headache: Theoretical problems. *Behav. Res. Ther., 16:* 249–261, 1978.
64. REEVES, J. L. EMG-biofeedback reduction of tension headache: A cognitive skills-training approach. *Biofeedback Self Regul., 1:* 217–225, 1976.
65. RYBSTEIN-BLINCHIK, E. Effects of different cognitive strategies on chronic pain experiences. *J. Behav. Med., 2:* 93–101, 1979.
66. SAINTSBURY, P., AND GIBSON, J. F. Symptoms of anxiety and tension and accompanying physiological changes in the muscular system. *J. Neurol., Neurosurg. Psychiatry, 17:* 216–224, 1954.
67. SARGENT, J. D., GREEN, E. E., AND WALTERS, E. D. The use of autogenic feedback training in a pilot study of migraine and tension headaches. *Headache, 12:* 120–125, 1972.
68. SARGENT, J. D., GREEN, E. E., AND WALTERS, E. D. Preliminary report on the use of autogenic feedback training in the treatment of migraine and tension headaches. *Psychosom. Med., 35:* 129–135, 1973.
69. SARGENT, J. D., WALTERS, E. D., AND GREEN, E. E. Psychosomatic self-regulation of migraine and tension headaches. *Semin. Psychiatry, 5:* 425–428, 1973.
70. SERES, J. L., AND NEWMAN, R. I. Results of treatment of chronic low-back pain at the Portland Pain Center. *J. Neurosurg., 45:* 32–36, 1976.
71. SILVER, B. V., AND BLANCHARD, E. G. Biofeedback and relaxation training in the treatment of psychophysiological disorders: Or, are the machines really necessary? *J. Behav. Med., 1:* 217–239, 1978.
72. STERNBACH, R. A. *Pain Patients: Traits and Treatment.* Academic Press, New York, 1974.
73. STURGIS, E. T., TOLLISON, C. E., AND ADAMS, H. E. Modification of combined migraine-muscle contraction headaches using BVP and EMG feedback. *J. Appl. Behav. Anal., 11:* 215–223, 1978.
74. SWANSON, D. W., FLOREEN, A. C., AND SWENSON, W. M. Program for managing chronic pain: II. Short term results. *Mayo Clin. Proc., 51:* 409–411, 1976.
75. SWANSON, D. W., MARUTA, T., AND SWENSON, W. M. Results of behavior modification in the treatment of chronic pain. *Psychosom. Med., 41:* 55–61, 1979.
76. SWANSON, D. W., SWENSON, W. M., MARUTA, T., AND MCPHEE, M. C. Program for managing chronic pain: I. Program description and characteristics of patients. *Mayo Clin. Proc., 51:* 401–408, 1976.

77. TURIN, A., AND JOHNSON, W. Biofeedback therapy for migraine headaches. *Arch. Gen. Psychiatry, 33:* 517–519, 1976.
78. TURK, D. C. Cognitive-behavioral techniques in the management of pain. In *Cognitive Behavior Therapy: Research and Application*, edited by J. P. Foreyt and D. J. Rathjen. Plenum Press, New York, 1978.
79. TURK, D. C., AND GENEST, M. Regulation of pain: The application of cognitive and behavioral techniques for prevention and remediation. In *Cognitive-Behavioral Interventions: Theory, Research, and Procedures.* edited by P. C. Kendall and S. D. Hollon. Academic Press, New York, 1979.
80. TURK, D. C., MEICHENBAUM, D. H., AND BERMAN, W. H. Application of biofeedback for the regulation of pain: A critical review. *Psychol. Bull., 86:* 1322–1338, 1979.
81. WEIN, K. S., NELSON, R. O., AND ODOM, J. V. The relative contributions of reattribution and verbal extinction to the effectiveness of cognitive restructuring. *Behav. Ther., 6:* 459–474, 1975.
82. WOOLEY, S. C., BLACKWELL, B., AND WINGET, C. A learning theory model of illness behavior: Theory, treatment and research. *Psychosom. Med., 40:* 379–401, 1978.

INDIVIDUAL PSYCHOTHERAPY FOR CHRONIC PAIN: INTRODUCTION

The next two chapters, on Individual Psychotherapy, deal with a topic which has received very meagre attention. Although literature abounds regarding the relationship of pain and anxiety, "illness behavior," and treatment by cognitive, relaxation and behavior therapies, there is not a single review paper to be found on the subject of Individual Psychotherapy in chronic pain, and it is a matter of some curiosity that in the foremost scientific journal, viz., "Pain," devoting itself primarily to the study of pain, not one paper on this matter has appeared to date.

Why is this so? Some pain syndromes are recognized as being a manifestation of psychiatric disorder, variously being considered a symptom of "hysteria" or a concomitant of depression or other psychiatric disorder. Individual psychotherapy is a common treatment for many mental disorders. Why is it then used with such parsimony and why this apparent lack of interest when it comes to treating pain?

Keeping in mind the inherent problems of treating chronic pain patients by individual psychotherapeutic methods, Dr. Bellissimo and Dr. Tunks consider a wide range of psychotherapeutic methods while Dr. Pilowsky and Dr. Bassett focus on dynamic psychotherapy for treating their pain patients. They recognize the problem of treating 'pain' by psychotherapy, because of the patients' 'somatic' view of the problem. They discuss appropriate timing in exploration of the emotional aspects of pain and careful selection of patients for individual psychotherapy. On the other hand, the benefits patients derive from individual psychotherapy are clearly demonstrated. Systematic research in evaluating individual psychotherapy for chronic pain deserves closer attention. In the meantime, however, the lesson to be drawn from these two chapters is that individual dynamic psychotherapy should be given serious consideration in the treatment of chronic pain.

8

Individual Dynamic Psychotherapy for Chronic Pain

I. PILOWSKY, M.D.
D. BASSETT, M.B.

Within the psychotherapeutic armamentarium available to the clinician lie a number of interventions which can provide varying amounts of relief to the patient. The theoretical perspective influencing such interventions varies from therapist to therapist, but on several issues there appears to be broad agreement (27). Firstly, chronic pain determined initially by predominantly somatic inputs can be conceptualized as producing emotional and behavioral sequelae. Secondly, psychological problems of one kind or another can be the major contributors to a pain experience, with its attendant illness behavior. Thirdly, there exist a large group of patients in whom there is a significant discrepancy between the objective evidence of disease and their illness behavior. Pilowsky (31, 33) has termed this clinical phenomenon "abnormal illness behavior." When these observations are considered as a whole, it is apparent that any approach to a patient with chronic pain must include a psychological perspective (32, 46).

In this chapter, we will focus upon those psychological interventions in chronic pain which involve one therapist treating one patient. Behavioral and cognitive therapy and biofeedback are considered elsewhere in this volume. For the purposes of definition, we consider psychotherapy to broadly include those professional interactions between a designated therapist and client, in which the major therapeutic technique is verbal interchange and the goal is change in the client. For the purposes of discussion, we will consider the forms of psychotherapy under the following headings: features common to psychotherapeutic approaches, psychodynamic psychotherapy, hypnosis and combined approaches. It is important to realize that the separate consideration of therapeutic approaches is purely for convenience, and the clinical management of a patient must always be that blend of interventions considered appropriate to each case.

Features Common to Psychotherapeutic Approaches

It is well recognized that within all forms of psychotherapy there are common features which provide a universal framework for psychological treatments (8, 21). The psychotherapies applied to the problem of chronic pain reveal further common features (25, 26, 37, 44, 45) which include the unambiguous communication of concern, tolerance of negative responses to therapy, patience, cognitive input concerning the relevance of the therapy, and some form of physical contact. Upon these basic requirements the specific components of each therapeutic maneuver will be built. It has been evident to us that success or failure in therapy with these patients rests heavily upon these basic requirements. In view of their importance, it seems reasonable to consider them in further detail.

COMMUNICATION OF UNAMBIGUOUS CONCERN

Chronic pain patients are particularly sensitive to perceived rejection. This probably has its roots both in personality factors which produce vulnerability to the development of chronic pain and in the events which often surround the chronic pain syndrome. Thus, Blazer (2) emphasized the narcissistic component of the personalities of chronic pain patients, while Engel (7) described the problems with interpersonal relationships and self-worth in the pain-prone patient. These patients tend to be preoccupied with their own plight and have often come to expect resentment and rejection from those around them. This conflicts with their need to obtain relief and support from their therapists, whom they often perceive initially as omnipotent. The result is anger and disillusionment, compounding their frequently poor self-esteem and self-critical attitude.

The approach of the therapist, then, must be such that it reflects a genuine concern for the patient's welfare and a desire to help. In doing so he must be aware that the patient will be more influenced by nonverbal and somatically orientated communications than by verbal or highly abstract communications. Thus, the experienced therapist will tend to enquire about the suitability of the chair offered the patient, ask about the current pain experience and encourage the patient to move about if he experiences difficulty in sitting through a long interview. Nonverbal cues such as the tone of voice and facial expression will also reflect the clinician's attitude to the patient.

TOLERANCE OF THE NEGATIVE COUNTERTRANSFERENCE

No matter how appropriate and clinically proper the therapist's attitude may be, the patient with chronic pain may, nonetheless, respond with cynical mistrust and resentment. It must be appreciated that many years of negative experiences may have preceded the interview and, as a consequence, trust cannot be expected to develop rapidly or, indeed, completely. Further, the thinly veiled (or not-so-veiled) hostility and the self-preoccupation of many of these patients frequently evokes feelings of hostility and resentment in the therapist. The result may be subtle changes in style, with the therapist giving covert messages of boredom or resentment.

For this reason the therapist must exert a considerable amount of restraint upon his own feelings and learn to tolerate the reticence with which some patients enter a therapeutic alliance. Often the patient will use the interaction as a test of the therapist's worth and will begin to trust and truly enter an alliance only after several sessions have elapsed.

PATIENCE

From the discussion thus far, it is evident that managing chronic pain patients demands that the therapist have the capacity to tolerate over periods of time the lack of gratification and positive feedback which must inevitably be the case with a patient who cannot relinquish the sick role. This is particularly true during the early stages of therapy when the major issues are "relevance" and "trust," with sometimes slow progression to full involvement in the treatment program. Indeed, even when participation is good, progress is often slow or incomplete after substantial effort.

COGNITIVE INPUT

It is essential in this context to provide the patient with a clear, readily comprehensible explanation of what the therapist believes is contributing to the patient's pain experience, and what he considers ought to be done. This contribution is often one of the most important ones the therapist makes, as it allows exchange of views and beliefs which may be vital to a productive alliance. Many patients respond to the proposal of a psychological therapy by inferring that their pain is considered imaginary or "in their head." If the therapist can negotiate these misconceptions, the way is open to establish a productive therapeutic alliance. It is also at this time that useful pragmatic advice and assistance can be given. It is, of course, easier to provide such information and advice in the context of a multidisciplinary pain clinic.

PHYSICAL CONTACT

It has been our experience that a somatic intervention of some kind is almost essential to the successful management of chronic pain (35). This is hardly surprising when it is recalled that the patient has chosen to express his discomfort in somatic terms and has presented asking for help with physical distress. The intervention need not be a major one in order to be effective and sometimes a brief physical examination, even one limited to the affected part, is sufficient to establish considerable trust. When the patient is being assessed and treated in the context of a Pain Clinic, the somatic approach to the patient is readily provided. It has also been our experience that some physical intervention is helpful while psychotherapy is in progress. This can take the form of regular physiotherapy or similar treatment. On no account should a clinician withhold a physical examination for which there appears an indication simply on the grounds that it may reinforce illness behavior. Such an approach can lead to serious diagnostic errors and, furthermore, tends to impede the psychotherapeutic process.

Psychodynamic Psychotherapy

PSYCHODYNAMICS OF THE PAIN EXPERIENCE

This conceptual framework derives its structure from psychoanalysis and offers a particularly useful approach with its emphasis on the interplay of biological and psychological forces. Pilowsky (34) has reviewed the psychodynamics of pain in some detail and only a brief outline will be included here. Brief case vignettes are included to illustrate the relevance of the various metapsychological perspectives or "views" of personality functioning.

The *dynamic view* emphasizes the part played by innate drives—such as sex, aggression and dependency. It is often apparent in clinical practice that a patient's pain is inextricably connected to one or more of these drives. The pain may serve as a means of releasing a drive in an acceptable manner which results in partial or complete gratification. It is important to appreciate that the use of pain as a mechanism to regulate or satisfy a drive which cannot be relieved more adaptively results in a disproportionate distribution of "psychic energy" (cathexes) toward the pain and away from other psychic functions. The result is often an impairment of routine activities and behaviors, which may become a problem in its own right and may be perpetuated by secondary gain.

Case History 1

Mrs. N. I. was a 57-year-old married woman who presented with pain in her back, abdomen, left groin and left leg. This began 12 months earlier when she slipped on a polished floor at her place of employment, a telephone exchange (which was about to be automated) in a small country town. She spent 4 months away from work but returned at her own request, with no appreciable improvement in her pain despite a variety of treatments (including traction, acupuncture, chiropractic manipulation and the use of minor analgesics). As her husband also worked and she did shift work, they met for an extended period only once every 3 weeks. He planned to retire in a year, and she intended to join him to travel around the country together in a trailer. These plans were in doubt now that she had constant pain.

She described her childhood as rather unhappy, with an alcohol-dependent father and a semi-invalided mother who had elephantiasis (filariasis) involving her left leg. She left school at age 14 to care for her mother and continued in this role until she married at age 21. When she returned from her honeymoon, she found her mother much less disabled and remaining so subsequently. She described her mother as a very difficult woman who could not get on with anybody. After her father died, she was often obliged to care for her mother but this caused conflict within her own family and she was faced with deciding where to place her loyalties. Her only sibling, a brother 7 years her junior, refused to have anything to do with his mother. Eventually the patient placed her mother in a nursing home and felt profoundly guilty for having taken this step. Two years before presentation, Mrs. I's mother died at age 84. There was an unhappy encounter with her brother at the funeral, and she did not feel that the relationship was in any way resolved.

When the patient was 11, she developed abdominal pain, but this was not diagnosed until she was 18; it was diagnosed as gall bladder disease with pancreatitis and was treated by cholecystectomy when she was 21. She saw a similarity between that experience and the current situation in which she felt that no one accepted that she had been in pain, leaving her feeling angry and resentful. Following in-patient psychotherapy, conjoint marital therapy and physiotherapy, she showed less depression and pain.

Comment. This case illustrates the association between anger, guilt and the development of chronic pain. A predisposing childhood experience is evident, while contemporary events, including her employment problems, marriage and bereavement, are clearly significant as precipitants. Her pain also provided an obstacle to her husband's plans which would inevitably have led to much closer contact between them.

Case History 2

Mr. N. was a 35-year-old married man who had suffered from right subcostal pain for the previous 18 years. He also recalled having abdominal pain as a child. When he was aged 15, he was told that the pain was "psychological" in origin, and he did not seek further help until 2 years prior to presentation when the pain became much worse. Despite thorough investigation, no relief for his pain could be achieved. He was, however, able to work and function as he wished despite the pain and believed that the etiology was emotional. He could also see that episodes of pain were clearly related to emotional disturbances.

His history revealed a childhood dominated by illness, with an attack of poliomyelitis at the age of 5 years which kept him in bed for 12 months and away from school 18 months. He regarded himself as being "always sick" until age 20, when he had a hemorrhoidectomy. He had an appendectomy at age 14 and also had sustained numerous fractures.

He was apprenticed as a printer but, once qualified, gave this up to become a real estate salesman. He married at age 20 and described his wife as quiet, introverted and lacking in confidence. They had suffered from marital problems for some time and were considering separation at the time of his presentation. Four years previously they had both made suicide attempts and both received psychiatric counseling. They had 2 daughters, aged 11 and 14, who were well.

He described his father as a man who drank heavily and gambled and had retired from his job as a stevedore 2 years earlier. He described his mother as extremely neurotic, insecure and lacking in confidence. He had found it impossible to live at home with her because she seemed to "fear everything." She dominated by constant overdramatization and frequent illness. He noted that she was "always afraid of death and disease."

During psychotherapy, it became evident that he linked pain with sexuality, and the possible relevance of homosexual feelings was explored. He was able to examine his feelings of shame, inadequacy and guilt surrounding his childhood, while approaching more slowly the association of pain with sexual feelings. Eventually he was able to discuss his homosexual feelings and touched briefly upon the association between anger and pain, which strengthened his acceptance of therapy. At the conclusion of his treatment, his pain had improved but not disappeared and he expressed gratitude for the help he had received.

Case History 3

Mrs. I. was a 29-year-old divorcee who presented with headache and neck and left shoulder pain, associated with intense paresthesia in her fingers. This followed a flexion-extension injury ("whiplash") of her neck in a motor vehicle accident while on her way home from work. She recovered after an 8-week convalescence, but the pain returned with greater severity after a second whiplash injury 16 months later (6 months prior to presentation). She suffered constant pain since then. Her major concern was the impact which her pain had had upon her social and sporting life, which were severely limited.

Her childhood was dominated by her parents' frequent arguments, culminating in their divorce. Her father was alive at the time of presentation but suffering from asbestosis and secondary chest infections. She said they had little in common. Her mother was also in poor health, with neck pain and hypertension; her mother attributed her pain to "lugging children around," and Mrs. I. said she avoided her because conversation consisted of "comparing neck notes." She described her mother as a domineering and difficult woman who often belittled her children.

The patient was the third of 4 children, and as a child used to withdraw from her family by reading. She left school midway through high school and took a variety of jobs.

At age 19 she married a policeman, and because of their shift work they did not see very much of each other. She considered it "a story-book marriage" and her husband as a "Prince Charming." After 5 years he left her and lived with another woman. They were divorced soon after, and she had difficulty coping with this experience. Despite the divorce, she remained very close to her in-laws and regarded her former mother-in-law as a substitute mother.

Two months prior to her presentation, her employer had been killed in an aircraft accident, resulting in a new person taking over his position. The company had changed considerably as a result, and she found all these events very unsettling. They added to her worry about her parents' health and about the compensation case surrounding her injury.

It was apparent that psychological issues were contributing significantly to her pain experience, and a course of brief psychotherapy was recommended.

The *structural view* places emphasis upon the functional divisions of id, ego and superego, as well as the body image, self-image and internal object representations which are integral components of the ego. The body image is built not only on a physical awareness of body parts but also on the person's unique emotional investment in its parts. It is the peculiar distribution of such investments in each individual which leads to differences in the "meaning" of injury, illness or pain between different people. Szasz (47) has developed these concepts further and suggests that the body image can be conceptualized as an "object" analogous to other living objects and that the individual may regard and respond to his body as if it were another person.

The superego has particular relevance to the pain experience since it is concerned with the role of internalized cultural values and expectations, with attendant shame and guilt when failure to meet these goals occurs. Pain is often closely associated with punishment and thus the development of superego functions. When inflicted pain during early development is great, a close association may develop in the child's mind between pain and punishment, with its associated guilt. This may develop as an expectation for pain to follow punishment or to substitute for it. In some individuals, excessive pain inflicted in childhood results in an introjection of these expectations, with persistent low self-esteem and masochistic personality traits. A similar effect can be observed when other noxious childhood experiences occur, and the same combination of hostility and poor self-image occurs.

Case History 4

Mrs. B. I. was a 53-year-old married woman who presented with pain in her neck radiating up into her head. The pain had begun 4 years earlier while she was pulling a heavy object from under a table. Her husband was in the hospital at the time after undergoing emergency open-heart surgery. She described him as a very selfish man who had no concern for her at all. This contrasted with her opinion of herself which was that she had done everything she could for him and did not complain, even when in great pain. He had retired on a pension and she was annoyed by his constant dissatisfaction with her housework. He blamed her for the heart attack which preceded his operation and she felt resentful that she could not even talk about the pain she was suffering. She complained that she slept poorly, but early morning wakening was not present.

Her husband was partially impotent but refused to seek help and had avoided sexual activity for several years. She was very angry about this and considered it yet "something else I have to do without." She relied very heavily upon her religious beliefs for support and was a regular church attender. One of her daughters provided her with considerable support, but she had little contact with her other 3 children (all from a previous marriage). Her husband maintained regular contact with his children from a previous marriage and left her feeling jealous of them as a result. She had some friends, but found her husband antagonistic to their visiting her at home.

Mrs. I. was the second of 4 children, with 2 sisters and 1 brother. Her father died when she was aged 3, leaving her mother to raise the family. Her mother did not remarry but relied upon Mrs. I. as the eldest daughter to help care for the other children. The eldest child, a male, was given a privileged position, as their mother believed men should be treated in this way. Mrs. I. said she had agreed with this. She was enuretic until aged 14, and menarche occurred at about this age. She had few boyfriends and was married at age 20 to a man with whom she had a most unhappy relationship. Despite this, she remained with him for 26 years "for the sake of the children." Soon after divorcing him, she had married her present husband.

Comment. This patient illustrates the association between chronic pain and hostility in relation to parents and parental figures. She also shows the tendency toward adopting a masochistic posture in close relationships.

The *adaptational view* is concerned with the coping and defensive maneuvers individuals employ to cope with stress. Here the use of ego defense mechanisms is paramount and the resulting effect upon conscious experience and behavior provides the variations observed among individuals responding to stress. In the context of disorder or injury, the behavior exhibited has been termed "illness behavior" (23). This behavior may be adaptive or maladaptive, with the latter being termed "abnormal illness behavior" (31). These behaviors can be classified (33) into those in which the motivation is predominantly conscious (e.g., malingering) and those in which it is mainly unconscious; those in which the focus is on somatic dysfunction and those in which it is psychological dysfunction; and those in which illness is inappropriately affirmed or inappropriately denied. The common forms of abnormal illness behaviors encountered in association with chronic pain are those in which the focus is somatic, illness is affirmed and the motivation is predominantly unconscious. When the patient manifests a preoccupation with illness and symptoms or a fear of disease, a hypochondriacal neurosis may be diagnosed. When the patient denies any preoccupation or fear but simply presents the pain and its consequences as a problem, a diagnosis of conversion neurosis is appropriate. In either case, the presence of dysphoria (depression or anxiety) may be denied or may be acknowledged and considered entirely as a consequence of physical illness. (The diagnosis can, of course, be made definitely only after the patient has been presented with a clear description of the therapist's view of the nature of the illness and the "appropriate" course of management to be adopted.)

Case History 5

Mrs. T. C. was a 37-year-old married woman with 2 children. She was receiving compensation payments for her pain which followed an incident at work in which she had slipped on a greasy kitchen floor. She explained that she had not reported the injury immediately, despite considerable pain, because she did not want to be called a "complainer." When she did seek help, she did not obtain relief for her pain and despite several attempts to return to work had been unable to persist with her employment. She had become increasingly mistrustful and cynical about doctors and their treatments. Her sleep was poor and dyspareunia interrupted her sexual activity.

Her previous health had been reasonably good, apart from an admission to the hospital for several days as an 8-year-old child. She also reported a deep venous thrombosis several years earlier and a tubal ligation.

She recalled a very close relationship with her father, whom she described in particularly glowing terms. He died when she was aged 12. Her mother was still alive and was described as being "more like a sister than a mother." Her mother remarried in the same year that the patient married.

She described a "happy" childhood with fond memories of her father and a close family, including her 2 siblings and mother. At age 14 she married a man 4 years older and noted that most of her family married very young. Their marriage was described as "special" to her, but, on questioning, she revealed that her husband had been unfaithful several times earlier in their married life. She now regarded these incidents as inconsequential and tended to idealize her husband. Her work record was particularly important to her as she believed she was regarded as a "good worker" and highly respected by her employers. It upset her to think that her employer had challenged her compensation claims, but she was even more concerned that she had been forced by her injury to give up work. She did not blame her employer for her injury but referred to it as "bad luck."

Comment. In this case the denial of anger toward authority figures was striking. She exhibited difficulty in tolerating this hostility and showed the use of reaction formation and illness behavior as coping strategies.

The Process of Psychodynamic Psychotherapy

Within this group of therapies, we include those which rely upon a body of theory derived from psychoanalysis and which attempt to use the relationship which develops between patient and therapist as a major therapeutic tool. It is convenient to divide the therapeutic styles into brief psychotherapy, extended psychotherapy and psychoanalysis. The differences between these include not only the time required but also the approach to therapy. Brief psychotherapy is usually considered to involve about 12 to 25 45-min sessions, although some therapists consider up to 50 sessions to be brief. Extended psychotherapy can be considered to include more than 20 (or 50) sessions, with no accepted limit. Psychoanalysis usually involves five 50-min sessions per week for at least several years. Perhaps the major differences, however, lie in the approach of the therapist in these sessions and the subsequent differences in the process of therapy itself. During brief psychotherapy the therapist is usually more active, with purposeful focusing upon certain predetermined areas of interest. The patient is encouraged to focus upon these areas and treatment goals are clearly delineated. The intrusion of unconscious material into the therapeutic relationship is interpreted immediately by the therapist, and insight is actively encouraged. Above all, reality testing is encouraged throughout the therapy, thus reducing the intensity of the transference. In contrast, extended psychotherapy is characterized by greater restraint upon therapist activity and less intense interpretation of transference phenomena. However, face-to-face contact is maintained, providing a reinforcement to reality testing. Psychoanalysis aims to intensify the development of transference by providing face-to-face contact, regression through recumbant posture and delay in interpretation of transference material.

As would be expected, the aims of these three techniques are different. Brief psychotherapy is usually focal in goals and attention, with definite agreement about the precise purpose of therapy before it begins. Extended psychotherapy is less focal, while psychoanalysis undertakes major personality reconstruction. Although transference has been focused upon here, other aspects of the interaction between patient and therapist are important. This is particularly true in brief psychotherapy where transference may not even be discussed in any way. The other components of therapy include suggestion, abreaction, manipulation, clarification and interpretation of defense mechanisms (1). Malan (19) has elegantly drawn together many of these concepts by referring to two "triangles of conflict": the first connecting unconscious feelings (or impulses), the defense mechanism and the accompanying anxiety; the second (derived from Karl Menninger, "The Theory of Psychoanalytic Technique") connecting the transference ("here and how"), a significant other ("current time or recent past") and a parent (usually "distant past").

Case History 6

Mrs. G. was a 32-year-old married woman with 3 children. She presented with a 5-year history of back pain, which had not been relieved by a laminectomy 12 months earlier. She recalled that the pain began while she was witnessing an argument between her eldest sister and brother-in-law. She said that this had reminded her of arguments between her parents many years before.

The pain had been "bearable" until 2 months prior to the laminectomy when an exacerbation followed the effort of pushing her car. She had been treated with psychotherapy during the previous year "for anxiety" and found the experience helpful. She was concerned, however, that the therapist might uncover things she could not cope with and was glad to terminate therapy.

Her developmental history was dominated by memories of a violent, alcoholic father who frequently beat her mother and her. She was the third of 5 children and did not feel close to her siblings. Her relationship with her eldest sister was particularly poor and she recalled that her sister was her father's favorite. She remembered a particular incident when, while arguing with her sister, she threw a milk bottle and cut her sister's foot quite badly. Her father was furious and called Mrs. G. a "killer."

Her menarche was at age 13 and she suffered from considerable dysmenorrhoea. She was sexually promiscuous as a teenager and was pregnant when she married at age 19. By then she considered she had "come to my senses" and described a very happy marriage subsequently. She insisted that the marriage was not entered into because of her pregnancy but had been decided upon before this was known.

At interview, she presented as an attractive woman who was visibly anxious and wept on several occasions. It was clear that psychological factors were contributing significantly to her pain experience and were derived from her traumatic early experiences, her relationship with her sister and the arrival of her daughter at an emotionally critical age. More specifically, she had been exposed to powerful, traumatic experiences as a child which resulted in her developing fragile self-esteem and considerable hostility toward important figures in her life. This was complicated by the introduction of sexual issues at a time when she was likely to have unconscious sexual impulses toward important males. The resulting guilt became an important contributor to her behavior and may have influenced the acting out of sexual impulses during adolescence. Her relationships with her mother (as a rival and recipient of her father's abuse) and her sister (as a rival and favorite of her father) were important, since she could not readily resolve these by the mechanism of identification. When she witnessed the argument between her brother-in-law and sister, her repressed anger and guilt were mobilized and neutralized by pain, possibly influenced by somatic inputs. During subsequent therapy she was able to recall an event which resulted in the aggravation of her pain, consistent with this formulation.

Therapy began with an explanation of the approach to be used, with emphasis upon her active participation. She accepted the principles of the therapy but was skeptical about its relevance to her pain. Throughout the first session and continuing into the second, she maintained an aggressive stance, with frequent questions and subtle criticisms. When this hostility was remarked upon, she denied it vigorously. Nonetheless, she became much less hostile and by the third session was talking freely about her early experiences and their relevance to her present problems. She began to use humor to reveal her anger and was able to recognize this fact. By the fifth session, it was apparent that positive feelings toward the therapist were coming to the surface, and these were commented on. She denied this as being relevant but did not change in her open and frank discussion. In the sixth session, she raised the experience of a very emotionally important involvement between her priest, another woman and herself. It appeared that the other woman had become openly very jealous of the good relationship Mrs. G. had with the priest and had caused problems to develop. This led to a discussion of the significance of triadic relationships for her and she herself made the connection to her own childhood. This proved to be an important session and her ambivalence to her father was explored in the next session. The subsequent session was relatively uneventful, although she raised the matter of her pain again and commented that although it was much better, "I think that's because of the injection I had" and not due to psychotherapy. Her apparent hostility was again remarked on and she again denied it.

During the following session she brought up the subject of triadic relationships and talked at some length about her sexual feelings toward her priest. She was able to reflect upon her guilt at this and talk freely about her attempts to cover it. The opportunity was taken to raise the topic of positive transference, which was discussed at some length. Notably it was possible to present to her the idea that she may have had mixed feelings toward the therapist and this may have been an important issue in other relationships. She could not accept this at the time but came to the next session reporting that several very significant events had occurred. It appeared that the previous day her car had broken down at a very inconvenient time, and she had become very angry with her husband. She had contacted him and told him so, only to be aware of intense feelings of guilt subsequently. She then recalled having felt equally angry with him the day (over a year previously) when she had pushed her car and her pain had become much worse. This realization left her emotionally very upset and she cried continuously for some time afterward. By the time she presented again she had talked it over with her husband and felt very much better. The remaining sessions were spent exploring the relevance of ambivalence to her and the role pain had played in expressing anger and guilt. Before terminating after 12 sessions, some time was spent discussing termination and it was decided that she might benefit from biofeedback-assisted relaxation training.

After therapy had been concluded, she was interviewed by an independent assessor and reported that her pain was very much improved and she felt generally very much better. She related this improvement to the injection she had received prior to psychotherapy and to the psychotherapy itself. She considered that the pain had improved considerably following the psychotherapy and felt better equipped to cope with her life's problems because of the therapy. This was confirmed by an independent interview with her husband.

Comment. This case history illustrated the contribution dynamic psychotherapy can make to the alleviation of chronic pain in some patients. Significantly, her pain was rarely discussed, and the context of the therapy was never questioned once begun.

Supportive Psychotherapy

It is convenient at this point to reflect upon that form of psychotherapy which aims specifically to support and strengthen the patient's own coping mechanisms. Here the emphasis is upon reinforcement of strategies the patient is already using, with no attempts being made to challenge defenses. The therapist is usually more active and positive, with maximal reality testing and encouragement. The time element is usually comparatively limited, with frequency and length of contacts varying enormously. The value of this approach is not to be underestimated and remains the bulwark of any therapeutic endeavor. This is never so evident as in the management of pain patients, where supportive psychotherapy is often the patient's major therapy.

The Efficacy of Dynamic Psychotherapy in Chronic Pain

The value of dynamic psychotherapy in the management of chronic pain has been recognized for some time (25–28, 36–38, 48). Despite this definite clinical impression, however, there is a dearth of empirical evidence supporting its efficacy in such patients (45). Outcome studies in dynamic psychotherapy are notoriously difficult (19) and their application to chronic pain is no exception. Among the reasons for this are problems in measuring outcome, achieving an adequate therapeutic alliance and choosing appropriate controls. Considering each in turn, the goal of therapy in such patients is difficult to define. Relief of pain provides a useful focus but is itself hard to measure. Further, it has been observed that a patient may appear very much brighter, happier and more active, without alteration in subjective pain reports. Psychodynamically, it appears perfectly reasonable that to relinquish the pain may itself be an enormous task (because of its ego defensive value), but considerable progress toward more mature coping strategies can be made without having to relinquish this. Thus when outcome is measured, many aspects of the patient's life-style and subjective satisfaction with treatment must be taken into account.

Case History 7

Mrs. B. was a 43-year-old married woman who presented with pain in her abdomen. The pain was described as constant with periods of exacerbation and had been present for 13 months prior to the patient's presentation. She had had an oophorectomy 6 months previously but this had failed to relieve her pain. Seven years previously a hysterectomy and unilateral oophorectomy had given relief of a similar pain. Her main complaint on presentation was that her pain had severely interrupted her life-style, which was previously very active.

She was the fifth of 5 siblings and described a close relationship to her parents. At school her academic performance was mediocre, but she took a very active interest in sport. This involvement continued after she left school, and she went on to participate extensively in sporting activities. As time progressed, she moved from participation to administration in sporting organizations and, until her pain began, she was very heavily involved.

A review of her sexual history revealed that she had her menarche at age 11, and it was associated with dysmenorrhea. She dated boyfriends from age 14 and married at age 23. She initially described the marital relationship as a good one, punctuated by relatively minor problems. However, she recalled that she was unable to have her own children because her husband had a low sperm count and she had "ovarian disease." Her husband was initially opposed to adoption, but they finally did adopt a boy and a girl.

She had worked in an office position for most of her married life but lost her job 2 months before presentation after an extended period of absence due to her pain.

During psychotherapy the patient rapidly progressed to examination of her feelings concerning her illness and the impact it was having upon her life-style. It became evident that she felt very distressed by having anything wrong with her body and was concerned that her pain might be with her indefinitely. This was compounded by her fear and revulsion at being dependent upon others and was aggravated further by her husband's irritation with dependent behavior. She explained that his mother had been an invalid for many years and he was very sensitive about this. She added that as the youngest child in her family she had learned to look after herself and not to depend upon others for her needs. To establish an identity for herself, she had felt the need to strive harder than most. She believed that her mother had tried to share herself evenly among her children, and Mrs. B. felt she never received as much attention from her mother as she needed.

As therapy proceeded, she focused more on her children and, in particular, on her son. She was concerned that he had poor self-esteem and appeared to be "getting involved with the wrong sort of company." It transpired that dyslexia had been a problem for him throughout his schooling and had contributed to his poor self-image and poor scholastic performance. She was now concerned that his employment prospects were poor and his problems would increase. These issues were discussed in the light of her own childhood experiences and she recognized her need to be the "perfect" mother. While exploring these areas, she came to consider the impact of having teenage children upon her view of herself and admitted to concern at her advancing age and failing physical prowess.

During the eighth session, she raised the subject of sexuality and revealed that she had recalled a traumatic incident during her childhood when one of her brothers had made a sexual assault upon her. She felt very angry and guilty about this incident and considered it might be relevant to her concern about having teenage children who were becoming more interested in sex. She was able to admit to some anger toward the therapist and to link this to her earlier experiences. Her hysterectomy and oophorectomies were seen to be relevant in this context, and she associated her loss of her sexual organs with her increased concern with sexual issues.

She became more relaxed in subsequent sessions and readily approached issues concerning her son and his behavior. The nature of adolescence was examined, and she was relieved to learn that much of her son's behavior could be understood in these terms. She was able, as well, to explore her feelings concerning these events and became much more comfortable with them. As her treatment drew to a close, she reviewed her progress and expressed intense satisfaction at what she had done. She believed her pain itself was unchanged but admitted that it was now much less of an issue in her life.

Comment. This case illustrates the possibility of improvement without pain reduction. The use of dynamic psychotherapy appeared effective, yet the pain could not be said to have improved. Despite this, the patient was very satisfied with her treatment.

Although psychotherapy is often considered appropriate in the management of chronic pain, these patients frequently resist entering into a meaningful therapeutic alliance (4, 12, 15, 36, 37, 40, 48). The reasons usually lie in difficulties with achieving trust in the therapist and with the presumed implications of psychological treatment. Patients often feel that they are being labelled as "mad" or "imagining their pain" and are slow to believe that the therapist accepts what they say. Indeed, patients will often readily acknowledge that they have labelled others suffering chronic pain in this way and have wondered from time to time whether they were themselves "imagining" the pain. This posture can be partly managed by combining psychotherapy with a somatic treatment (e.g., physiotherapy), even if the latter is nonspecific in its aims (35, 37, 48). If the patient is assessed and treated by a multidisciplinary pain clinic, this will also tend to help by promoting obvious somatic intervention and presenting the psychotherapist in juxtaposition with other somatically orientated therapists (35, 37).

In addition, the pain clinic context provides support for the approach a particular therapist is taking, thus dealing with the problem of nagging doubts over the possibility of overlooking pathology.

The choice of experimental controls in studying this form of therapy is not easy. The major problems are related to the complexity of a therapy whose precise characteristics will inevitably vary from therapist to therapist.

While it is easy to find a comparison group, it is often difficult to deal with the problems caused by the duration of treatment and the length of exposure to the motivated therapist. One can compare the therapy to some other therapies, but large differences remain in the rate of progress expected and the appropriate outcome measures (19). It is probably not surprising, therefore, that in our survey of the literature we have been unable to find a single controlled study of dynamic psychotherapy in the treatment of chronic pain. There is, however, anecdotal evidence, and it is our personal experience that such therapy has a place in the management of the majority of patients.

Maruta et al. (17) report a study in which 31 patients presenting with low back pain were treated with a variety of individual and group psychotherapies, combined (as deemed appropriate) with antidepressants, minor tranquilizers and physiotherapy. Eight patients scored 3 or 4 on the four-point outcome scale, while cooperation was scored as 3 or 4 in 13 patients. The difficulty in interpreting these results, with such varied treatments, is obvious. Hasenbush (9) reported the case of a 72-year-old man with chronic pain and drug abuse. He was prescribed amitriptyline, an activity program and reduced drug and alcohol intake, while receiving brief psychotherapy (9 sessions). The patient's wife had 4 concurrent sessions with the therapist's wife (a social worker). Considerable improvement in the patient's activity, mood, drug and alcohol consumption, and marital relationship was observed. Unfortunately, there is no clear documentation of the outcome of the patient's pain. Other workers report the use of group psychotherapy (20), but controlled studies are absent.

The Application of Dynamic Psychotherapy to Chronic Pain: Details of Therapy

The use of dynamic psychotherapy in chronic pain rests heavily upon the realization that the pain itself should not be the prime focus. Merskey and Spear (28) emphasize the subjective sense of fear and concern which accompanies the pain and suggest that this should be the prime focus of psychotherapy. The pain remains an important symptom, but, as Knoll (12) explains, few of these patients are good subjects for intensive psychotherapy. He recommends approaching emotional issues slowly and carefully, confronting the patient's resistance to therapy and lack of trust. Sometimes the pain constitutes a critically important defensive mechanism for the patient, and removal or attempted removal is inevitably highly anxiety provoking (3, 12).

It is our practice to emphasize cognitive input early in treatment during the "negotiation" phase and to choose an appropriate style of therapy as time progresses. The focus is upon those problems which the patient has identified during the assessment period, and the subject of pain is rarely introduced by the patient after the early sessions are completed. As has been mentioned previously, clear emphasis is placed upon the pain and its somatic aspects during assessment. It is our belief that it is this early emphasis upon the pain which allows trust to develop more rapidly and progression to psychological issues to occur more easily. Pinsky (36) recognizes the usefulness of this approach. He maintains that these patients tend to verbalize feelings with difficulty and choose to express distress more in somatic language. If this is recognized and communicated to the patient early, the patient himself will frequently shift attention away from pain and onto interpersonal and emotional issues. McCranie (22) has explored this aspect further and has reformulated "conversion pain" (a form of hysterical conversion neurosis) as the expression of emotional distress in somatic form. He maintains that the traditional analytical formulation of conversion as a partially effective defensive maneuver to cope with unconscious conflict presents a negative view of the patient's distress. He also recommends aiming therapeutically at the distress and the exploration of its origins. Blazer (2) conceptualized this problem in terms of narcissism and proposed that chronic pain patients tend to have a narcissistic personality structure. As a consequence, they respond to stress with primitive defense mechanisms (denial, projection, somatization) and demonstrate an upsurge in narcissistic interest in their bodies. This chimes with the suggestion that pain constitutes a threat to the body schema (42).

Blazer (2) argues further that the patient, having regressed in the face of a threat to his body integrity, looks to parental figures (e.g., doctors) for omnipotent relief. When relief is not forthcoming, he responds with rage but is unable to expose this easily because of the inherent fear of rejection. To combat this, Blazer recommends being alert to this hostility and meeting it with tolerance and patience. He emphasizes the role of the therapist in reassuring the patient that the therapist appreciates the seriousness of the problem. Here we would add that the therapist can help dismantle the patient's fantasies of the therapist's omnipotence by pointing out the real limitations of therapy, as well as its strengths. Indeed, by emphasizing the limitations of therapy the therapist is covertly reassuring the patient that the defensive apparatus will not be prematurely dismantled. Blazer concludes that psychotherapy is facilitated by activities which enhance the patient's sense of self-control, such as biofeedback, self-hypnosis and relaxation exercises.

Hypnosis

Considerable interest has arisen in the use of hypnosis in the management of pain (10). Although used clinically very extensively, most of the systematic studies have involved experimentally produced pain. This has left a significant deficiency, as with many other treatment modalities (45). The anecdotal evidence is considerable, however, and Elton et al. (6) report a study which provided some systematic evidence of the efficacy of hypnosis in the relief of chronic pain. In this study, 50 patients suffering from chronic pain in a variety of anatomical sites were randomly allocated to hypnosis, biofeedback, placebo and behavioral psychotherapy. The study was complicated by the fact that all patients received a number of background treatments, including rational-emotive therapy and assertiveness training. At the conclusion of treatment, outcome was measured on a series of parameters, and hypnosis and biofeedback were found superior to the other treatments. No statistical analysis was included, and it appeared from the graphs presented that the hypnosis and biofeedback groups showed initially higher baseline measures.

In a study of hypnosis and EMG biofeedback in the management of chronic pain, Melzack and Perry (24) found that while combined treatment gave significant improvement in 60% of patients, hypnosis alone did not. No control group receiving no active treatment was used. It was significant that in neither of the two studies mentioned were subjects divided or selected into those who were good hypnotic subjects and those who were not. Hilgard and Hilgard (11) point out that only about 20% of subjects are highly responsive to hypnosis in this context, and one wonders what difference selection might make in clinical studies. Schlutter et al. (43) report a study in which hypnotic analgesia was compared with EMG biofeedback and EMG biofeedback plus relaxation training. They found no difference between these treatments, and all produced significant pain relief.

The approaches used during hypnosis vary from therapist to therapist, but relief of anxiety, altered cognitions and imagery are common features. The use of hypnosis has been greatly extended by the use of autohypnotic techniques (11, 41) which allow patients to extend the duration and contexts of treatment extensively. The mechanisms involved have not been fully clarified, but Hilgard (10) suggests that cerebral laterality in the processing of sensory information may be responsible. He refers to the differences observed between overt and covert cognitive responses which illustrate a dissociation in information processing.

Combined Psychotherapy

Thus far our attention has been focused upon individual psychotherapy. In practice, however, it is frequently appropriate to offer several different therapies simultaneously. This has been well recorded with behavioral and related treatments (5, 13, 29, 30, 39) as well as hypnosis (6). Legalis (16) reported 2 cases in which brief dynamic psychotherapy was combined with biofeedback to the distinct advantage of the patients. This is in keeping with the opinions we have already raised and the advice of Blazer (2) concerning combination of psychotherapy with somatically oriented therapies. Lambley (14) reported 1 case in which dynamic psychotherapy was combined with assertiveness training and presented evidence of the additive effect of these therapies. The inference from all these studies and our clinical experience is that combined therapies have considerable merit, but research is required to delineate more precisely the situation in which their effect will be greatest and most predictable.

REFERENCES

1. BIBRING, E. Psychoanalysis and the dynamic psychotherapies. In *Psychiatry and Medical Practice in a General Hospital*, edited by N. Zinberg. International University Press, New York, 1964.
2. BLAZER, D. G. Narcissism and the development of chronic pain. *Int. J. Psychiatry Med., 10(1):* 69–77, 1980.
3. CASTON, J., COOPER, L., AND PALEY, H. W. Psychological comparison on patients with cardiac neurotic chest pain and angina pectoris. *Psychosomatics, 11(6):* 543–550, 1970.
4. COBB, S., AND BONNER, F. J. Psychiatric considerations. In *Pain. Its Mechanisms and Surgical Control*, edited by J. C. White, and W. H. Sweet. Charles C Thomas, Springfield, IL, 1955.
5. DANIELS, L. Treatment of urticaria and severe headache by behaviour therapy. *Psychosomatics, 14:* 347–357, 1973.
6. ELTON, D., BURROWS, G., AND STANLEY, G. Hypnosis in the management of chronic pain. In *Hypnosis, 1979*, edited by G. Burrows, D. Collison, and L. Dennerstean. Elsevier, Holland, 1979.
7. ENGEL, G. Psychogenic pain and the pain-prone patient. *Am. J. Med., 28:* 899–918, 1959.
8. FRANK, J. Common features of psychotherapy. *Aust. N.Z. J. Psychiatry, 6:* 34–40, 1972.
9. HASENBUSH, L. Successful brief therapy of a retired elderly man with intractable pain, depression and drug and alcohol dependence. *J. Geriatr. Psychiatry, 10(1):* 71–88, 1977.
10. HILGARD, E. Hypnosis and pain. In *The Psychology of Pain*, edited by R. Sternbach, Raven Press, New York, 1978.
11. HILGARD, E., AND HILGARD, J. *Hypnosis in the Relief of Pain.* Kalfman Inc., Los Altos, CA, 1975.
12. KNOLL, R. Psychoanalysis and pain. In *Pain: Research and Treatment*, edited by B. Crue. Academic Press, New York, 1975.
13. LAKE, A., RAINEY, J., AND PAPSDORF, J. Biofeedback and rational emotive therapy in the management of migraine headache. *J. Appl. Behav. Anal., 12:* 127–140, 1979.
14. LAMBLEY, P. The use of assertive training with psychodynamic insight in the treatment of migraine headache: A case study. *J. Nerv. Ment. Dis., 163(1):* 61–64, 1976.
15. LARGE, R. Chronic pain and the psychiatrist. *Aust. N.Z. J. Psychiatry, 48(1):* 113–115, 1978.
16. LEGALIS, C. Biofeedback and psychotherapy. *Semin. Psychiatry, 5:* 529–533, 1973.
17. MARUTA, T., SWANSON, D., AND SWENSON, W. Low back pain patients in a psychiatric population. *Mayo Clinic Proc., 51:* 57–61, 1976.
18. MALAN, D. The outcome problem in psychotherapy research. *Arch. Gen. Psychiatry, 29:* 719–729, 1973.
19. MALAN, D. *Individual Psychotherapy and the Science of Psychodynamics.* Butterworth, London, 1979.
20. MARBACH, J., AND DWORKIN, S. Chronic M.P.D., group therapy and psychosomatics. *J. Am. Dent. Assoc., 90:* 827–833, 1975.
21. MARMOR, J. The nature of the psychotherapeutic process revisited. *Can. Psychiatr. Assoc. J., 20:* 557–565, 1975.
22. McCRANIE, J. Conversion pain. *Psychiatr. Q., 47:* 246–257, 1973.
23. MECHANIC, D. *Medical Sociology.* Free Press, New York, 1968.
24. MELZACK, R., AND PERRY, C. Self-regulation of pain: The use of alpha feedback and hypnotic training for the control of chronic pain. *Exp. Neurol., 46:* 452–569, 1975.
25. MERSKEY, H. Psychiatric aspects of the control of pain. In *Advances in Pain Research and Therapy, Vol. 1*, edited by J. J. Bonica, and D. Albe-Fessard. Raven Press, New York, 1976.

26. MERSKEY, H. Psychiatric management of patients with chronic pain. In *Persistent Pain*: *Modern Methods of Treatment*, edited by S. Lipton. Grune & Stratton, New York, 1977.
27. MERSKEY, H. The role of the psychiatrist in the investigation and treatment of pain. *Res. Publ. Assoc. Res. Nerv. Ment. Dis.*, *58*: 249–260, 1980.
28. MERSKEY, H., AND SPEAR, F. *Pain*: *Psychological and Psychiatric Aspects*. Balliere, Tindall and Cassell, London, 1967.
29. MITCHELL, K. Note on treatment of migraine using behaviour therapy techniques. *Psychol. Rep.*, *28*: 171–172, 1971.
30. MITCHELL, K. A psychological approach to the treatment of migraine. *Br. J. Psychiatry*, *119*: 533–534, 1971.
31. PILOWSKY, I. Abnormal illness behaviour. *Br. J. Med. Psychol.*, *42*: 347–351, 1969.
32. PILOWSKY, I. The psychiatrist and the pain clinic. *Am. J. Psychiatry*, *133*: 752–756, 1976.
33. PILOWSKY, I. A general classification of abnormal illness behaviours. *Br. J. Med. Psychol.*, *51*: 131–137, 1978.
34. PILOWSKY, I. Psychodynamic aspects of the pain experience. In *The Psychology of Pain*, edited by R. Sternbach. Raven Press, New York, 1978.
35. PILOWSKY, I. Abnormal illness behaviour and sociocultural aspects of pain. In *Pain and Society*, edited by H. Kosterlitz, and L. Terenius. Verlag Chemie, Weinheim, 1980.
36. PINSKY, J. Psychodynamics and psychotherapy in the treatment of patients with chronic intractable pain. In *Pain*: *Research and Treatment*, edited by B. Crue. Academic Press, New York, 1975.
37. PINSKY, I., AND MALYON, A. The eclectic nature of psychotherapy in the treatment of chronic pain syndromes. In *Chronic Pain*: *Further Observations from the City of Hope National Medical Center*, edited by B. Crue. Medical and Scientific Books, New York, 1979.
38. RANGEL, L. Psychiatric aspects of pain. *Psychosom. Med.*, *15(1)*: 22–37, 1953.
39. REEVES, J. EMG-biofeedback reduction of tension headache: A cognitive skills-training approach. *Biofeedback Self Regul.*, *1*: 217–226, 1976.
40. RITTERHOFF, D. Psychiatric evaluation and feasibility of psychiatric therapy. *J. Occup. Med.*, *17(10)*: 656–657, 1975.
41. SACERDOTE, P. Teaching self-hypnosis to patients with chronic pain. *J. Human Stress*, *4(2)*: 18–21, 1978.
42. SCHILDER, P. *The Image and Appearance of the Human Body*. International University Press, New York, 1950.
43. SCHLUTTER, L., GOLDEN, C., AND BLUME, H. A comparison of treatments for prefrontal muscle contraction headache. *Br. J. Med. Psychol.*, *53*: 47–52, 1980.
44. STERNBACH, R. *Pain Patients. Traits and Treatment*. Academic Press, New York, 1974.
45. STERNBACH, R. Clinical aspects of pain. In *The Psychology of Pain*, edited by R. Sternbach. Raven Press, New York, 1978.
46. STERNBACH, R. Psychological techniques in the management of pain. In *Pain and Society*, edited by H. W. Kosterlitz, and L. Y. Terenius. Verlag Chemie, Weinheim, 1980.
47. SZASZ, T. *Pain and Pleasure*, Basic Books, New York, 1957.
48. WEBB, W. The therapy of psychosomatic pain. *Curr. Psychiatr. Ther.*, *18*: 73–84, 1978.

9

Individual Psychotherapy for Chronic Pain

ANTHONY BELLISSIMO, Ph.D.
ELDON TUNKS, M.D.

"There are no procrustean beds in which the patient should be fitted. The therapist must formulate an independent therapeutic rationale and working hypothesis for each patient undertaking psychotherapy" (23, p. 35).

Current literature in individual psychotherapy reflects the continuing presence of a number of competing systems of psychotherapy. Within this context, there are a number of themes and basic principles which are important in psychotherapy with the chronic patient. The first theme focuses on the common elements of psychotherapy (7, 12, 13, 15, 29, 43). Frank (13) summarizes this theme by stating, "for beneath the babble of conflicting claims, all schools of psychotherapy share certain features that combat a state of mind of most of their patients, regardless of their specific symptoms." He goes on to label the "state of mind" as "demoralization." The second theme focuses on specific factors affecting the process and outcome of psychotherapy: the impact of the therapist, the technique, and the characteristics of the patient (18). The third theme is the urgency for the development of therapeutic strategies based on specific knowledge of problems such as chronic pain, sexual disorders, and psychosomatic conditions (24). The final theme is that of integration. Goldfried (16, 17) suggests that this integration may be possible around common "principles of change" that are empirically based.

Debates about the objectives and the process of psychotherapy are also to be found in the literature, with some authors attempting to elaborate these (14, 16, 17, 24). Thus, Karasu (23) lists the objectives of psychotherapy as consisting of any or all of the following: 1) achieving relief when in crisis, 2) obtaining the reduction or elimination of symptoms, 3) moving toward the strengthening of defenses and integrative capacities, 4) reaching a resolution or rearrangement of conflicts, and 5) achieving personality changes leading to more adaptive functioning. In discussing the process of psychotherapy, Bellak (4) emphasizes the learning process. He sees the need for learning to be linked to 1) a sound theory of personality, 2) hypotheses directed at the development of psychopathology, and 3) interrelated propositions, developed from 1 and 2, which direct the patient to restructure maladaptive patterns into adaptive ones.

An urgent need to develop more specific and more effective psychotherapeutic procedures is recognized. This results from the growing zeitgeist in the general field of psychotherapy (16, 17) and also from the general awareness that truly effective management of such problems as chronic pain has not yet been achieved. The rationale for specificity has been recently expressed by Karasu and Bellak (24) who state that, "the more specific and better conceptualized the hypotheses concerning a given form of psychotherapy and its treatment, the more effective a therapy is likely to be." The idea that a particular clinical strategy may not be appropriate for all problems in all circumstances has been expressed by many writers. In 1967 Paul (36) emphasized the point by stating, "what treatment, by whom, is most effective for this individual with that specific problem, and under which set of circumstances?"

The Special Case of Chronic Pain

The commitment to therapeutic strategies based on specific knowledge of unique problems has resulted in specialized therapies such as sex therapy (30) and psychotherapy for "borderline patients" (25), for example. However, several factors seem to have delayed the development of specialized techniques in the individual psychotherapy of the chronic pain patient. The puzzle of the pathogenesis of chronic pain syndromes has yet to be solved, and already the emerging model of chronic pain is very complex. The individual with chronic pain presents the clinician with a unique subjective experience that has cognitive, affective and sensory aspects. In addition, knowledge and management of the chronic pain problem are significant only if they take into account the patient's personal background and ongoing life circumstances, which include the patient's family and health care system. In the midst of such complexity, the psychotherapeutic operation involves more factors than can be accommodated within a single therapeutic model, and a focus on variables such as psychodynamic conflict, stress and disturbed interpersonal relationships leads to only limited benefits from each. No single technique appears to suffice.

THE PSYCHODYNAMIC PERSPECTIVE

Individual psychotherapy based on psychoanalytic principles has had very limited impact in the area of chronic pain, notwithstanding psychoanalytic literature on the subject (5, 6, 8, 11, 22, 27, 44). The suggestion has been made that the unsatisfactory results of attempts to apply this therapy with chronic pain patients are due in part to inappropriate goals (for example, the complete relief of pain) and poor selection of patients. Tunks and Merskey (45) indicated that a more appropriate goal for dynamic psychotherapy of pain patients may be the exploration of the meaning of the pain and the role that pain plays and had played in the affective and interpersonal economy of the patient. They pointed out that the patients must be appropriately "psychologically minded" to benefit from therapy. These patients often lack this characteristic and need much help to examine the broader social and environmental context of their pain and dysfunction. Further, they are not just bothered by unpleasant affects and ineffective defenses but are beleaguered by dependency on agencies, by lack of income, and by uncertainties about their future. Therapies which have a narrow intrapsychic focus must necessarily be supplemented by or coordinated with programs that deal with the larger issues: vocational assessment, occupational retraining programs, social counseling and assistance.

Another difficulty is that chronic pain patients often are still in receipt of various medical, surgical and anesthesiological treatments, and, therefore, confusion about the meaning of their pain may easily arise, compounding psychotherapeutic tasks. The psychotherapist may have to become a coordinator of messages in order for the patient to maintain a consistent attitude toward treatment.

Moreover, the psychological approach is frequently unpalatable to pain patients. They often do not do well in traditional psychotherapeutic settings because they perceive the problem as medical and as distinct from a psychological issue. To be in receipt of psychotherapeutic treatment, it may be necessary to visit the office of a psychiatrist or a psychiatric outpatient department where the patient reference group or treatment setting may be seen as being at variance with how they want themselves to be perceived. It has been suggested that, wherever possible, psychologically oriented therapies should be carried out in the setting and by therapists most compatible with the nature of the chief complaint (20, 28).

Pain patients perceive themselves as being afflicted and requiring cure. In contrast, the usual expectations for successful participation in psychotherapy are such things as readiness in divulging psychological material (or free association), willingness to think and talk in psychological categories, having a focus for psychological change and insight, etc. The style of the therapist tends to be nondirective or passive in the expectation that the patient will be productive. This sort of general style may be inappropriate for a patient who expects active intervention as an adequate sign of therapist interest and competence (41).

The esoteric language of traditional psychotherapy may have less relevance to the majority of pain sufferers. Efforts have been made to make the psychotherapeutic method relevant. For example, Stafford-Clark (40) and Pos (37) suggested that pain symptoms might be considered as analogous to obsessional symptoms, and Waldman (47) suggested that pain be considered a fiction (a mode of conduct subject to will and responsibility relating to sick role and its interpersonal meaning). The problem again is that these efforts still have not provided a language in which the patient can be engaged in a process of therapeutic persuasion without resort to the esoteric language that may be unacceptable to the chronic pain patient. This is in addition to the distinct possibility that the arguments of the papers may be fallacious. Papers which have stressed nonspecific elements of therapy, like the work of Frank et al. (14), are perhaps more relevant to the special case of pain treatment. Unfortunately, whereas the concepts delineated by this group do provide a framework for discussion of the effective elements in psychotherapies, they do not provide good guidelines for mounting specific management in individual cases.

The psychodynamic spectrum of psychotherapy is quite complex and varied, ranging from classical psychoanalysis to object-relations to ego psychology. However, all writers share the belief that human activity is the end result of internal dynamic forces and that intervention should focus primarily on these internal forces rather than on environmental variables. Thus the thrust of psychodynamic psychotherapy can be summarized by the following theses:

1. A patient's symptoms and problems are meaningful creations of the patient, but the meaning may be more or less outside his awareness.

2. Treatment involves helping the patient achieve awareness within the context of a confiding and safe relationship with the therapist.

HOPE IN THE NEW APPROACHES

In recent years the area of "behavioral medicine" has emerged as a potential source of concepts and treatment strategies for chronic pain. In this context, operant conditioning approaches as well as more broad behavioral therapy methods have been used for the management of chronic pain. Specific procedures have included biofeedback, autogenic training, and jacobsonian deep muscle relaxation training. These procedures are effective by reducing anxiety (48, 49). In the area of individual treatments, there has been an influential movement in the development of "cognitive psychotherapy." This provides an alternative to the interpretative traditional analytic stance. (Further discussion is found in Chapter 7 by Cameron.) Such methods may be more easily adapted to the problem of chronic pain.

There is a discrepancy in the literature between the amount of attention given to the topic of biofeedback as a clinical tool for the control of chronic pain and the very limited empirical evidence supporting its intrinsic efficacy (1, 46, 51). A few studies that appeared in the literature demonstrated the possibility of developing techniques for the treatment of chronic pain using biofeedback principles (9, 33). These developing biofeedback applications may vary in focus from the training of patients to increase activities which direct attention away from pain, to focus on reducing and/or controlling anxiety and tension, or to focus on cognitive factors such as mastery and sense of control (31).

Recent developments in therapy using behavioral procedures have emphasized the role of cognition. The focus has been in part on individual differences in cognition: the way individuals interpret and/or organize events. How the individual's interpretation and organization act as determinants of behavior problems can be studied and used to restructure behavioral change. The importance of cognitive factors in the area of pain has been identified in the literature (34, 42). Recently Weisenberg (48, 49) has emphasized the importance of cognitive factors with respect to pain assessment and management.

Perhaps there is not yet a coherent body of theory that could be called "cognitive psychotherapy," but rather there is a group of related approaches. These approaches have mainly been explored and developed in experimental settings, with preliminary application being made to pain problems (Chapters 11 and 12). The pivotal concepts are as follows: The thought processes that accompany behavior change are behaviors too, albeit covert. (Access to these behaviors is by some form of inquiry and response.) Understanding the thought patterns and restructuring them may provoke some change in that behavior to which the thought is linked. In maladaptive or problematic behavior or in symptoms, several patterns of thought tend to be frequently encountered: unwarranted assumptions regarding the significance of the event, generalization, "catastrophizing," and attributions that make the problem insoluble or render the individual helpless. Of these, the two most important patterns may be those of making unwarranted assumptions (requiring educational programs for pain patients) and of "catastrophizing" (which may be a personal characteristic of poor responders versus good responders in any form of treatment) (39). Successful coping tends to be frequently associated with opportunities for advance preparation for the stressful event, opportunities to preview it so that expectations are more consonant with reality, and opportunities for practicing various coping methods such as physical relaxation strategies, distracting imagery, and imagery that alters the significance of the threat. These strategies must be practiced consistently and must be selected purposefully by the subject. The general clinical application of "cognitive psychotherapy" concentrates on two general approaches: "self-monitoring" and exploration of "internal talk" and rehearsal and practice of coping strategies.

Modeling as an agent for behavioral change has been studied for a number of years (2, 38), but the specific application of the modeling concept to pain has been systematically explored more recently by Craig and Best (10).

Deliberate application of these ideas to chronic pain is as yet no more than anecdotal but may prove to be a valuable element if not a treatment strategy in itself (Chapter 12).

Hypnosis for pain has been reviewed extensively and utilized for many years. A consensus does seem to emerge, however, that this specific psychotherapeutic method is not applicable to all patients (21, 35). There is some debate whether hypnosis ought to be considered a special form of communication (52), a technique for tapping or manipulating various levels of consciousness (21), or an interaction depending heavily on perceived expectations and beliefs probably mutually shared (3). Certainly, no physiological cerebral state can be identified as corresponding to an hypnotic "trance": in this sense the trance cannot be defined physiologically to exist the same way that sleep can. It is probably a peripheral issue, however, to argue whether any of these conflicting positions are more correct. From a pragmatic point of view, it appears that hypnosis can be effectively combined with other treatment modalities for reducing anxiety and enhancing the sense of personal control, but it probably is not a sufficient treatment in its own right for most chronic pain problems. The theoretical models employed simultaneously with the hypnotic methods might be taken from either general psychology, transactional analysis, or other theories of human behavior (50). As with other specific psychotherapy methods, it seems that only a minority of patients are "appropriately psychologically minded" to do well with the method. One deficit, at least with some forms of application of hypnosis, is that it tends to project a message of the therapist enacting some cure on the passive patient. Recently Spanos et al. (39) studied the relationship of cognitive strategies to hypnotic susceptibility and to suggestions for analgesia. They found that the hypnotic trance induction was itself not shown to be necessary, but that high hypnotic susceptibility, the personal characteristic of not being a catastrophizer, and receiving simple suggestions for analgesia all seemed to have a positive influence in producing the desired experimental effect.

MANAGEMENT VERSUS TREATMENT

Frank and his colleagues (14) have extensively studied the "Effective Ingredients of Successful Psychotherapy" and published their findings. If their findings can be generalized, one would note a general applicability not only to various psychotherapies but also to other forms of management, such as behavior modification programs, placebos, interdisciplinary treatment package programs, back education classes, etc. To summarize, the nonspecific essentials for effective behavioral change appear to be: 1) Therapist and patient involved in therapeutic contact. Therapist and patient are behaving in culturally appropriate ways. 2) A rationale exists and is shared by both the patient and healer, but the healer is an expert in the use of this rationale both to explain the disorder and distress and to suggest means to overcome it. 3) A therapeutic focus is identified and agreed upon. 4) Motivation to change exists and may be further aroused by the therapist's behavior, the treatment context and the treatment rituals. 5) A ritual which is based on and consistent with the rationale is employed and actively involves the patient, providing him at least symbolically with a sense of mastery. 6) After a period of working through his problem, the patient is allowed to apply his new skills in his natural environment where he previously encountered difficulty, and he is discharged.

Another general management issue is noted in that many chronic pain programs have a psychosocial thrust which affects most of the operation carried out, but the patients themselves may not be involved in an easily recognizable psychotherapy. They are managed, however, according to the principles drawn from psychotherapy: for example, maximizing appropriate defenses, teaching coping strategies and working through adaptational problems in the context of relationships (see chapter 12 by Baptiste and Herman).

Principles of Psychotherapy and the Problem of Chronic Pain

In the Dahlem Workshop on Pain and Society (26) the group reported on principles of pain management and expressed, among others, the following conclusions: "Those treatments seem to work best which possess or require high activity, high visibility, high contact, and high apparent relevance." The application of individual psychotherapy to chronic pain may achieve a higher level of efficacy if the above conditions are present.

The individual psychotherapeutic intervention for a specific patient must arise from an understanding of his pain as a complex, personal and interpersonal adaptation to distress and other stress. It must take into account specific knowledge of the unique problem of pain (as a motivation, sensation, and cognition). Thus, for example, one must use the available information about the variables that appear to influence perception of pain. Some of the important factors have been discussed by Melzack and Chapman (32). These include: 1) attention, 2) anxiety, 3) depression, 4) rewards and secondary gains for taking and maintaining a "chronic pain posture" and 5) cultural and developmental factors associated with the expression and/or experience of pain. "Personality" structure and "previously-acquired adaptive skills" should be added to this list. Considering the foregoing, the psychotherapeutic process with chronic pain patients should focus on achieving the following objectives: 1) help the patients take an active role in their own treatment, 2) focus on an adaptive and informed (cognitive) orientation in the understanding of the complex pain problem, 3) assist the patient to develop coping strategies and 4) shift the treatment focus toward more adaptive general "life-management" strategies.

Characteristics of high activity, visibility, contact and relevance appear to be met easily in clinics especially devoted to chronic pain where educational programs, group therapies and behavioral modification programs can be mounted in the context of a multidisciplinary setting which may be more palatable to chronic pain patients and with a reference group that may be more acceptable, i.e., a group of other chronic pain patients rather than psychiatric patients. In this it is important to consider the family and environment of the chronic pain patient in the intervention.

CASE EXAMPLES

The 3 cases presented here are not meant to represent comprehensive treatment of people with chronic pain. They are meant to highlight the variety of psychological intervention strategies and styles of individual psychotherapy for chronic pain patients. As a group, the 3 cases show in a practical, clinical way some of the issues discussed in this chapter. These are actual treated cases and represent both success and failure.

Mrs. J. T.

This 31-year-old married woman had a 1½-year history of Reiter's syndrome, including symptoms from polyarthritis, iritis, and stomatitis, and she suffered from diarrhea and anemia. She was referred for assessment of depression. In the initial interview she admitted that her life had changed significantly since her illness. Previously, she had been a national level athlete and had had her own crafts business. Now she was unable to compete or even to participate in the sports she had previously enjoyed; she suffered a lack of motivation and energy and a loss of self-esteem. There were classical signs of depression, including insomnia with early morning awakening and diurnal mood variation, but there were no signs of psychosis.

In the initial interview she described her family of origin as having been ideal and suppressed a number of most unpleasant facts about her rearing. She had been a middle child of three, and because of her father's government job the family moved frequently. She had married an independent business man 8 years previously and they had chosen to have no children. Also about 8 years ago, she had undergone a nephrectomy because of hydronephrosis.

The patient presented herself as being distressed strictly on account of arthritis and her inability to carry out her previously active life-style. Antidepressants were offered. In follow-up, she complained of extreme side-effects at even miniscule doses of medication. However, there was much conversation regarding the nature of her thinking while depressed which tended to perpetuate her depressed feelings. It was evident that she "catastrophized" and projected herself into helpless and useless self-perceptions and behaved as if others might have the same evaluation of her.

She still would not take more than miniscule amounts of antidepressants but was interested in talking about her disease, her responses to it, and her social responses; she became interested in regaining some "control" over some important areas in her life. She reasserted that her marital relationship was solid and that relationships with her parents were positive. Ten weeks after her first visit, a new symptom of anxiety verging on terror presented. This had begun episodically but now was dominating her day and was coloring everything she thought or did. She found this paradoxical because it had recently been explained to her that her disease was now in remission except for some dryness of eyes and discomfort on exercise, and her business had been going well. Yet, she was suffering nightmares and was constantly seeking reassurance from her husband and friends. She wondered "whether people were getting fed up with her" or whether she was "bringing this on herself by a bad attitude that was making her ill." It was learned that at that particular time her husband was away for a week of work in another city. She still refused antidepressants.

At the next interview her husband was seen conjointly with her. He questioned whether his wife's reaction to medication was due to her previous nephrectomy or was due to a "psychological distaste for medication." He felt that his wife was not conveying her feelings completely.

In further regular conversations, she reported her relief that she was not required to take medications. One particular issue that was discussed involved feelings of irritability and tension that impaired her in her waiting on clients in her shop. At times she could respond crossly and now approached each client with rising apprehension, which she attempted to control by avoiding clients as much as possible. She came to realize that her apprehension was based on the exaggerated and generalized fear that she would be cross with everyone and recognized that her avoidance only served to perpetuate her fear. After beginning to monitor her thoughts and report them in her conversations with the therapist, she felt much improved and relieved. She also concluded that her physical health had previously had much to do with her self-esteem and that, deprived of it, she had assumed a less valued and "less-in-control" attitude as well with others. As she continued to monitor her thinking patterns, her negative self-statements diminished.

Prior to her illness she had enjoyed yoga which had given her a sense of mastery over her mind. During her depression, however, her concentration had not allowed her to practice, and now she found herself unable to return to these good feelings. A few sessions of hypnosis allowed her to successfully return to her yoga.

Despite bouts of influenza and an episode of herpes zoster, she felt after 4 months that she was able to carry on without help from the therapist. After a hiatus of 5 months, she again asked for help. She stated that she had done well until recently while attending a convention sponsored by her husband. Halfway through the day, she suddenly felt overwhelmed and panicky and ran from the hotel to return home. The following week, while seeing friends off at the airport and while contemplating a trip of her own a few months hence, the same panic returned and now was generalizing to all crowd or travel situations. A tentative formulation was proferred in terms of anxiety as a reaction to an unfamiliar environment, complicated by her escape responses which reinforced the anxiety and subsequent generalization. A scheme of cognitive self-monitoring and gradual in vivo desensitization was suggested.

She followed the suggested routines but, in addition, in subsequent sessions revealed much new material. She had a rich deam life which she recorded and discussed. Through it, she revealed her life as a child. Her father had abused pills and alcohol and when intoxicated was particularly prone to sexually molest her. (Hence her fear of medication of any kind.) After molesting her, he either would be remorseful and overcompensate or would ignore the issue completely. Mother was no help; a silent suffering "victim" who never fought or complained, but whose long-suffering was probably painful for everyone. Neither parent provided an adequate role model for dealing with anger. J.T. sometimes felt annoyed that mother did not leave father but could not express this because she ambivalently accepted mother's verdict that father "was sick," and mother certainly seemed to be above reproach. She felt ambivalently toward her changeable father. She thought maybe she loved him, but, considering the explicit sexual nature of her father's attention, that was dangerous too. (Making it more complicated, father some years later had undergone a conversion and apologized to J.T. for his misdeeds and swore off all drugs. Now there was obvious tension between her parents, which J.T. avoided.)

As a young adult, before and after marriage, she had gone through a chaotic time of angry promiscuity, feeling the compulsion to seduce men but having only contempt for them. She eventually had revealed this to her husband, talked about her anger, and ceased feeling the anger or the need to continue this pattern.

While still a child, J.T. had discovered that father admired physical vigor, and she had a "tomboyish" style and excelled in sports, much to his delight. By accident, she also discovered that "being ill" exempted her from parental and, particularly, paternal obligations and gave her warm attention unconditionally. A pattern developed in which she would press herself to excel but, if feeling less than a match for the task, she would quickly endorse symptoms, even factitious ones. This pattern had continued even into her marriage and into her relationship with the therapist; she recognized that she had in the first 4 months of therapy reconciled herself to not being obligated to excel and had then discontinued therapy. Attending her husband's conference, not as a star nor as a business woman but just as his wife, she said she suddenly developed "symptoms," and these had also brought her patient status again with the therapist.

Therapy was pursued using more of a dynamic focus, elucidating the libidinal, affectional and oedipal themes and their interrelations. The dream content reflected marked changes from anxiety to self-control and confidence during the course of therapy. Self-monitoring was still carried on to effectively eliminate the episodically anxious feelings or nightmares. After 1 year from the initial visit, she was discharged as asymptomatic and content that she was obligated neither to be sick nor to excel.

Comment. It should be noted that this patient was not "psychologically oriented" during first encounters. She was, however, oriented for an intervention based on a relationship and in the course of a number of months was able to move toward a more "insightful" dynamic focus. The therapy of J.T. underlined the need for a flexible style, shifting from cognitive-behavioral, to information processing (hypnosis), to interactional, to psychodynamic. The therapist was active on several counts—as a coordinator of information regarding the significance and status of her disease, offering strategies (cognitive-behavioral therapy), acting as a hypnotist, and generally keeping an active style in the dynamically oriented portion of therapy. Opportunities for mastery and the necessity for self-control were maximized throughout.

Mr. J.M.

This 49-year-old married man had suffered a motor vehicle accident 1 year previously, with a spinal cord injury which resulted in a Brown-Sequard syndrome, including pain and dysesthesias on the right side of the body and motor deficits on the left. Additionally, he suffered a sense of nervousness, loss of confidence, and inability to make decisions. Prior to his accident, there was no nervous complaint, although he had always been an obsessive and meticulous individual, and he had worked 30 years for the same employer.

No marital problems were described and there were no children. However, his wife was observed to be a timid and dependent individual who received most of her cues from him as to how she should respond. He had determined that she should not seek employment.

His childhood was described in bland terms. A period of alcohol abuse had ended 3 years previously when he began to attend Alcoholics Anonymous.

The initial management included attendance at the pain control classes, T.E.N.S., and functional assessment carried out by Occupational Therapy. Interviews were usually held conjointly with his wife. In the interviews, his style was loquacious and mildly argumentative, and he engaged in long embellished and monotonous discourses, which it seemed had always been characteristic of him. In groups (pain control classes) he used defenses of isolation, intellectualization and rationalization to neutralize any suggestions that might imply that he ought to change. Reports from the occupational therapist verified that his permanent neurological deficits were such as to make even a sedentary job difficult.

The one positive feature of his participation in the program was an enthusiastic endorsement of relaxation exercises. Therefore, the therapist involved him in a program of EMG biofeedback, to build on relaxation skills, and this was combined with a cognitive-behavioral approach which he found palatable.

In discussions among members of the pain team, his problem was formulated in psychodynamic terms (accepting, naturally, the medical and environmental issues as significant). His obsessive style had always hidden any sense of vulnerability or impotence and had previously served him well at work. His defenses, which had been more or less successful, had been further mobilized by his injuries and attendant insecurities. He would respond to therapist interventions as if they were commands or criticisms and would either argue or avoid them by noncompliance. Therapists concluded that insight-oriented therapy would continue to be rejected, but that his basic defenses were not bad and could be somewhat reorganized in a "less expensive" way.

A treatment strategy was adopted which was based on a relaxation task. He was asked to learn this task and then find ways to generalize it to his everyday situation. Despite some initial anxiety about taking such responsibility on himself, he devised a game of imagery which allowed him to relax and applied this to various situations. A great improvement in self-esteem resulted, his pain became less, and his self-confidence increased. He did not, however, attempt to return to work, and he received a disability pension.

Comment. This case illustrates the use of psychodynamic principles in guiding treatment. The patient himself, "not psychologically oriented," was oriented to a cognitive-behavioral style of problem solving. The net result was that the Pain Team made their plan in one language but did their various therapies in language that was more palatable to the patient. The conceptual framework guiding the whole operation could be seen as mobilizing the nonspecific factors in psychotherapy (14).

Mr. J.B.

Mr. J.B. was a 49-year-old single man who had chronic pain trauma Guillain-Barre polyneuropathy 10 years earlier. His physical and emotional functioning had been at the disabled level for the majority of this time, and his complaint of pain was great. He had a great fear that his polyneuropathy would return, and he would, for example, avoid walks, because if he began to tire and feel weak, he would be overcome with panic that he was having a recurrence. He became involved in individual psychotherapy after admission to the Pain Clinic.

He was the eldest, having a younger sister and brother. Father had left for military service when J.B. was 5 years of age and he remembered resenting it when father told him "look after the ladies while I'm gone" (mother and sister)—indeed, what about his own feelings, he thought! Mother was unfaithful and financially successful during father's absence. When father returned 8 years later, a long battle ensued. Mother was clever, self-centered and dramatic, dressed like a 1930s movie star and insulted all males. Father was ineffectual. Mother finally walked out on the family during a dramatic altercation on a Mother's Day "with the kids' cards sitting on the table." Shortly after, he was sexually molested by a strange male and later had great difficulty coming to terms with his latent homosexual feelings.

His male relationships were always perceived as tenuous because he feared being abandoned, but he was very successful in business.

His polyneuropathy had developed in a fulminating and life-threatening manner after a mild infection, and he spent time on a respirator in a rehabilitation center. He began to reject affectionate overtures by male intimates because he felt worthless. With difficulty he returned to work, but remembered that "one day someone asked 'How are you?' and that day I stopped saying 'Fine, thank you'." He recalled how, since then, he had allowed everything and everybody to slip away from him, stopped working and felt incapable of resuming independence. He came to the point of recognizing his responsibility for the attitude as to whether he should be "fine" or not, accepting that he would have residual dysesthesias and some motor weakness permanently. The complication was that, by now, his family had drifted apart; he was a middle-aged unattached and unemployed homosexual, very isolated and easily demoralized. He progressed only during Pain Clinic active treatment and regressed on discharge. The assistance of vocational rehabilitation agencies was insufficient support to allow him to progress, and he drifted back to his original state.

Comments. This patient illustrates the importance of the context of the problem. Therapists felt strongly that J.B.'s failure depended much on the lack of stable and sufficient social support. This lack was aggravated by a lifelong tendency to regard his interpersonal relationships as tenuous and, therefore, to let them go too easily. The fact that the Pain Clinic was situated in the Rehabilitation Centre, and that the pain program was oriented toward behavior modification, rekindled in him his lifelong feeling that duty came before his own needs. This in turn complicated his attitude toward members of the pain team who felt that he ought to be able to do something on his own. This had reopened the childhood experience in which he had felt himself insufficiently loved or deserving of appreciation. Accordingly, he had withdrawn to illness, which now legitimized being looked after by a general practitioner.

Conclusions and Guidelines

In spite of the complexity of the various competing conceptual models, some basic principles defining therapeutic change are in the psychotherapeutic literature (16, 17). These guidelines for psychotherapeutic management seem to have evolved from the ongoing interplay of theoretical orientation, clinical experience, and research knowledge (16, 17, 26). The concepts underlying these guidelines include: 1) the primacy of the patient-therapist relationship in any intervention; 2) the therapeutic value of structured new experiences that may be learned or even taught in therapeutic situations; 3) a focus that recognizes the areas of cognition and observable behavior as well as that of affect, and 4) the adoption of a therapeutic stance characterized by a high level of activity, contact and relevance.

Some guidelines as they apply to chronic pain can be further developed as follows:

1. Pain can be conceptualized as a potent affect, analogous to "signal anxiety." On this basis, rationale can be developed for treatment and patient education using the familiar structure of the psychoanalytic models.

2. The therapist assumes a role that might be described as "coach" or "tutor." This role emphasizes the therapist's interest in guiding and urging the patient to try new ways of thinking and behaving. This stance does not simply replace more conventional therapist-to-patient relationships but rather amplifies them. The core of the therapist-patient relationship remains intact, allowing the patient to "transfer" stereotyped patterns of relating to significant others from the past to the present and with the help of the therapist to experience awareness and achieve a corrective experience.

3. The "ecological" context is the framework in which the problem is considered and dealt with. However, the therapists highlight the developmental and sociocultural issues so that the patient achieves a more adaptive perspective about himself, others, and the interactions linking them. Direct attention is given to contextual information to help the patient develop appropriate sets of expectations. This can be achieved, in part, by directing the patient to explore the antecedents and consequences of patterns of behavior and feelings.

4. Attempts are made to shift attention from symptoms, where there is an opportunity to teach some "self-control," as in biofeedback.

5. Whenever possible, the focus will include problems in living, downplaying the symptom of pain itself.

6. Wherever appropriate and especially where progress is occurring, strategic shifts in theoretical model and therapist posture may occur, for example, from operant, to supportive, to dynamic conceptualization.

7. Despite the importance of an interpretive analytical focus, a cognitive-behavioral approach may often be more practical. Thus, current experiences can be structured in such a way that the patient may try new adaptive strategies and apply them to old problems. These structured situations can

take the form of actual interactions devised both inside and outside the psychotherapeutic context and, apart from providing mastery in their own right, provide important symbolic and analogical mastery experiences as the therapeutic relationship is "worked through."

8. An overall rationale for problem formulation and intervention must be available, particularly in multidisciplinary settings and in pain clinic package programs. These broader conceptual frameworks will provide a rationale accounting for both medical and behavioral issues as well as a basis for educational activity based on relationship aspects of the therapeutic situation.

REFERENCES

1. ANDRASIK, F., AND HOLROYD, K. A. A test of specific and nonspecific effects in the biofeedback treatment of tension headache. *J. Consult. Clin. Psychol., 48:* 575–586, 1980.
2. BANDURA, A., AND WALTERS, R. H. *Social Learning and Personality Development.* Holt, Rinehart and Winston, New York, 1963.
3. BARBER, T. X. Measuring hypnotic-like suggestibility with and without hypnotic induction. *Psychol. Rep., 16:* 809–844, 1965.
4. BELLAK, L. Once over: What is psychotherapy? *J. Nerv. Ment. Dis., 165:* 295–299, 1977.
5. BERENT, I. Original sin: "I didn't mean to hurt you, mother"—a basic fantasy epitomized by a male homosexual. *J. Am. Psychoanal. Assoc, 21:* 262–284, 1973.
6. BERNSTEIN, A. E. A psychoanalytic contribution to the etiology of "back pain" and "spinal disc syndromes." *J. Am. Acad. Psychoanal., 6:* 547–556, 1978.
7. BOWLBY, J. The making and breaking of affectional bonds: II. Some principles of psychotherapy. *Br. J. Psychiatry, 130:* 421–431, 1977.
8. CASTON, J., COOPER, L., AND PALEY, H. W. Psychological comparison of patients with cardiac neurotic chest pain and angina pectoris. *Psychosomatics, 11:* 543–550, 1970.
9. CLARKE, N. G., AND KARDACHI, B. J. The treatment of myofascial pain-dysfunction syndrome using the biofeedback principle. *J. Periodontol., 48:* 643–645, 1977.
10. CRAIG, N. G., AND BEST, J. A. Perceived control over pain: Individual differences and situational determinants. *Pain, 3:* 127–135, 1977.
11. ENGEL, G. L. Psychogenic pain and the pain prone patient. *Am. J. Med, 26:* 899–918, 1959.
12. FRANK, J. D. Common features of psychotherapists and their patients. *Psychother. Psychosom., 24:* 368–371, 1974.
13. FRANK, J. D. Mental health in a fragmented society: The shattered cyrstal ball. *Am. J. Orthopsychiatry, 49:* 397–408, 1979.
14. FRANK, J. D., HOEHN-SARIC, R., IMBER, S. D., LIBERMANN, B. L., AND STONE, A. R. *Effective Ingredients of Successful Psychotherapy.* Brunner/Mazel, New York, 1978.
15. GARFIELD, S. L. Basic ingredients or common factors in psychotherapy. *J. Consult. Clin. Psychol., 41:* 9–12, 1973.
16. GOLDFRIED, M. R. Toward the delineation of therapeutic change principles. *Am. Psychol., 35:* 991–999, 1980.
17. GOLDFRIED, M. R. (Ed.), Special Issue: Psychotherapy process. *Cognit. Ther. Res., 4:* 271–306, 1980.
18. GOMEZ-SCHWARTZ, B., HADLEY, S. W., AND STRUPP, H. Individual psychotherapy and behavior therapy. *Ann. Rev. Psychol., 29:* 435–471, 1978.
19. HALEY, J. *Uncommon Therapy: The Psychiatric Techniques of Milton H. Erickson.* Norton, New York, 1973.
20. HENKER, F. O. Diagnosis and treatment of nonorganic pelvic pain. *South. Med. J., 72:* 1132–1134, 1979.
21. HILGARD, E. R. The problem of divided consciousness: A neodissociation interpretation. *Ann. N.Y. Acad. Sci.,, 296:* 48–59, 1977.

22. HOPWOOD, M. A case of severe psychogenic pain. *Guy Hosp. Rep., 114:* 325–327, 1965.
23. KARASU, T. B. General principles of psychotherapy. In *Specialized Techniques in Individual Psychotherapy*, edited by M. T. B. Karasu and L. Bellak. Brunner/Mazel, New York, 1980.
24. KARASU, T. B., AND BELLAK, L. (Eds.) *Specialized Techniques in Individual Psychotherapy*. Brunner/Mazel, New York, 1980.
25. KERNBERG, O. Technical consideration in the treatment of borderline personality organization. *J. Am. Psychoanal. Assoc., 24:* 795–829, 1976.
26. KOSTERLITZ, H. W., AND TERENIUS, L. Y. *Pain and Society*. Verlag Chemie, New York, 1980.
27. LUBORSKY, L., AND AUERBACH, A. H. The symptom-context method: Quantitative studies of symptom formation in psychotherapy. *J. Am. Psychoanal. Assoc., 17:* 68–99, 1969.
28. MAI, F. Management of "psychosomatic" problems in clinical practice. *Can. Med. Assoc. J., 114:* 684–686, 1976.
29. MARMOR, J. Common operational factors in diverse approaches to behavior change. In *What Makes Behavior Change Possible?*, edited by M. A. Burton. Brunner/Mazel, New York, 1976.
30. MASTERS, W. H., AND JOHNSON, V. E. *Human Sexual Inadequacy*. Little, Brown, Boston, 1970.
31. MEICHENBAUM, D. Cognitive factors in biofeedback theory. *Biofeedback Self Regul., 1:* 201–216, 1976.
32. MELZACK, R., AND CHAPMAN, R. Psychological aspects of pain. *Postgrad. Med. J., 53:* 69–75, 1973.
33. MELZACK, R., AND PERRY, C. Self-regulation of pain: The use of alpha-feedback and hypnotic training for the control of chronic pain. *Exp. Neurol., 46:* 425–489, 1975.
34. MERSKEY, H., AND SPEAR, P. G. *Pain: Psychological and Psychiatric Aspects*. Balliere, Tindall, and Cassell, London, 1967.
35. ORNE, M. T. Mechanisms of hypnotic pain control. In *Advances in Pain Research and Therapy, Vol. I*, edited by J. J. Bonica. Raven Press, New York, 1976, pp. 717–726.
36. PAUL, G. Strategy of outcome research in psychotherapy. *J. Consult. Psychol., 31:* 109–119, 1967.
37. POS, R. Psychological assessment of factors affecting pain. *Can. Med. Assoc. J., 111:* 1213–1215, 1974.
38. SCHACHTER, S., AND SINGER, J. Cognitive, social, and physiological determinants of emotional state. *Psychol. Rev., 69:* 379–399, 1962.
39. SPANOS, N. P., RADTKE-BODORIK, H. L., FERGUSON, J. D., AND JONES, B. The effects of hypnotic susceptibility and suggestions for analgesia, and the utilization of cognitive strategies on the reduction of pain. *J. Abnorm. Psychol., 88:* 282–292, 1979.
40. STAFFORD-CLARK, D. Psychosomatic implications of obsessive-compulsive disorders and their resemblance to certain types of central pain. *Guy Hosp. Rev., 114:* 209–222, 1965.
41. STEINMULLER, R. The use and abuse of psychiatry in dealing with pain patients. *Psychiatr. Q., 51:* 184–188, 1979.
42. STERNBACH, R. A. *Pain: A Psychophysiological Analysis*. Academic Press, New York, 1968.
43. STRUPP, H. On the basic ingredients of psychotherapy. *Psychother. Psychosom., 24:* 249–306, 1974.
44. SZASZ, T. S. The nature of pain. *Arch. Neurol. Psychiatry, 74:* 174–181, 1955.
45. TUNKS, E., AND MERSKEY, H. Psychiatric treatment in chronic pain. In *Behavioral Problems and the Disabled*, edited by D. Bishop. Williams & Wilkens, Baltimore, 1980, pp. 238–271.
46. TURK, D. C., AND MEICHENBAUM, D. H. Application of biofeedback for the regulation of pain: A critical review. *Psychol. Bull., 80:* 1322–1338, 1979.

47. WALDMAN, R. D. Pain as fiction: A perspective on psychotherapy and responsibility. *Am. J. Psychother.*, *22:* 481–490, 1968.
48. WEISENBERG, M. The regulation of pain. *Ann. N.Y. Acad. Sci.*, *340:* 102–114, 1980.
49. WEISENBERG, M. Pain and pain control. *Psychol. Bull.*, *84:* 1008–1044, 1977.
50. WILLIAMS, D. T., AND SINGH, M. Hypnosis as a facilitating therapeutic adjunct in child psychiatry. *J. Am. Acad. Child Psychiatry, 15:* 326–342, 1976.
51. YATES, A. J. *Biofeedback and the Modification of Behavior.* Plenum Press, New York, 1980.
52. ZEIG, J. K. (Ed.) *A Teaching Seminar with Milton H. Erickson.* Brunner/Mazel, New York, 1980.

FAMILIES AND CHRONIC PAIN: INTRODUCTION

The next two chapters are devoted to the important area of family functioning. Family psychological theory and therapy are in fact substantially developed, but the application to families with members who suffer chronic pain has been somewhat late. Yet the "family approach" is evidently relevant, if only in that chronically ill individuals influence the dynamics of their families' functioning. Beyond this, the question arises whether family dynamics are implicated in the genesis of chronic pain. Dr. Mohamed addresses this issue, drawing on his own experience as well as some available literature. Because of the relative paucity of research up to this point, much of the evidence is necessarily anecdotal and clinical. A little more is known about the factors within the family that might perpetuate chronic pain. With this, Dr. Mohamed sketches the beginning of a workable, clear model. Part of this model is the perspective that the family can be considered as the unit of treatment. Lately, more attention is being given to the role of the spouse and, indeed, distress of the spouse in the case of the chronically ill family member, and these insights complement the psychiatric and behavioral literature on chronic pain.

Dr. Waring builds on this perspective in describing and illustrating the assessment and the treatment of families, using a different conceptual framework. Specific attention is given to "cognitive family therapy," which promises to be clinically effective and productive as an investigative tool for work with chronic pain.

The foundation laid by the two chapters, being based on practical clinical experience with families of chronic pain patients, offers hope to the clinician and avenues for exploration to the researcher.

10

The Patient and His Family

S. MOHAMED, M.D., F.R.C.P.(C)

Numerous studies in the literature have examined extensively the importance of psychological factors such as affect, motivation, attention, cultural background and personality as determinants of pain tolerance, the expression of pain, and complaints of pain in chronic pain patients (2, 10, 11, 14). Chronic pain has also frequently been a presenting complaint in patients with psychological illness and somatic complaints (18).

It is, however, surprising that until recently the role of family dynamics and marital dynamics has had little impact on the study of predisposing, precipitating or perpetuating variables in most chronic pain research and theories. Only in the past few years have health care practitioners realized that even chronic pain can be understood and treated with a family system perspective (6, 7, 9, 13, 16, 17). If the family operates as a system to enlarge or to maintain the pain problem, then the family needs to be treated to bring the pain problem under control. As a result, programs have been developed which integrate family oriented and behavioral treatment programs for chronic pain, with much better outcomes than previous individual based treatments (6, 7, 17).

Monographs on chronic pain from a psychological perspective by Merskey and Spear (11), Sternbach (14), Fordyce (3) and others have mentioned the chronic pain patient's psychological difficulties and the effect of these difficulties on the spouse and the family of the patient. The chronic pain patient becomes depressed due to loss of health, loss of enjoyable activities, loss of income and loss of capacity to fulfill previous roles as spouse and family member. These losses also profoundly affect the patient's spouse and family, who in turn experience depression and helplessness and respond with pain-reinforcing behavior (2, 10, 11, 14). Further, there is evidence that marital maladjustment and family dysfunction can play an important role in the selection of chronic pain as a symptom and in the perpetuation of chronic pain problems in at least a significant proportion of chronic pain patients (13, 16).

Liebman et al. (9) were the first to focus on family therapy for children presenting with chronic abdominal pain. Since then, Waring et al. (15-17) (see also Chapter 11) have used conjoint marital and family cognitive therapy with good success in the treatment of adult chronic pain patients.

This chapter, therefore, will review recent clinical and research evidence that implicates the role of the family in regard to predisposing, precipitating or perpetuating variables in chronic pain patients.

Definition of a Family

For the purpose of this chapter, a family will be defined by a marriage and all the subsequent additions or deletions to this dyad over the family life cycle. We will also differentiate between two distinct family groups. Family of origin will refer to the families of adult patients in which the patient grew up but which he has now left. A nuclear family will refer to both adult and child patients and their current families with whom they live. Finally, we will also refer to adult patients' current marital relationships.

In this discussion we will be describing correlations of marital and family maladjustment with chronic pain and discussing these factors as precipitating and, more importantly, as perpetuating factors and not generally in terms of causality.

A deficiency of social bonds may play a causative role in nonpsychotic emotional illness (12, 16, 17). However, chronic physical symptoms of obscure etiology may also contribute to disturbing social relationships. The social relationships may also be influenced by illness rather than disease and by abnormal illness behavior and/or sick role as opposed to the symptom itself. It remains for future empirical research to address the question of causation.

The Family as an Etiological Factor in Chronic Pain Syndrome

The role of family as an etiological factor was first observed by Freud, who found an increased prevalence of pain problems in patients and their respective families. Since then, it has been supposed that the family of origin may influence pain threshold, pain tolerance, pain complaints and/or the sick role (2, 11, 14). The literature reveals that pain-prone patients come from large families, that firstborn in families are often less tolerant of pain, and that complaints of pain are positively correlated with the experience of family members who also had pain (1, 10, 13).

Waring (15) hypothesized that pain experience may be turned into a complaint of pain due to the psychological significance of pain (conscious and/or unconscious) to a "significant other."

Mohamed et al. (13) demonstrated a positive correlation between a group of depressed patients with chronic pain as the primary symptom and a history of past pain problems and pain problems in their families of origin, the pain occurring in corresponding locations.

In summary, there is, therefore, some tentative evidence to suggest that family dynamics play an important predisposing role in some chronic pain patients. However, it cannot be determined if the correlations in the parental families are due to genetic factors or to specific family dynamics such as identification, imitation, modeling or operant conditioning since the latter also occur in spouses and their families.

The Role of Family in the Perpetuation of Chronic Pain Syndrome

THE CURRENT NUCLEAR FAMILY

Minuchin (12) found that the families of children with psychosomatic symptoms, such as anorexia nervosa, asthma, diabetes and chronic pain, demonstrated a number of clear family interactional characteristics including: 1) rigidity, 2) overprotectiveness toward the ill member, 3) poor problem-solving capabilities, and 4) overinvolvement or enmeshment with one another. Liebman et al. (9) describe a successful therapeutic program combining behavior modification and family therapy in 10 children with psychogenic abdominal pain. They comment that these children's pediatricians were drawn into a position of overinvolvement by parents. While the absence of control groups, confounding of outcome by using several treatment strategies, and absence of reliable outcome measures require reservations regarding the validity of outcome, the study is the first clinical report of the successful use of family therapy in chronic pain.

Recently Hudgens (6) has described a behavioral model of family involvement in the treatment of adult chronic pain patients with successful outcome.

Another significant study is that of Khatami and Rush (7) using modalities of symptom control, stimulus control and social system intervention in treatment of outpatients with chronic pain who had not responded well to treatments previously provided. Social system intervention consisted of direct instructions to family members to modify the positive and negative reinforcers for pain behavior, or structured family therapy. The therapist gave direct instructions to family members to provide interpersonal reinforcement (attention, concern or lack of attention), depending on whether the patient demonstrated pain behavior (e.g., complaining, helplessness, overdependent attitudes) or autonomous, responsible behavior (e.g., doing housework, working, self-care). In family therapy the therapist also functioned as a boundary-maker, separating parent from child subsystems. Each of the components of the treatment package resulted in therapeutic change. Generally, these improvements were maintained at 6-month and 1-year follow-ups. This study was consistent with the notion that chronic pain is maintained by a combination of interpersonal and intrapersonal factors.

The family characteristics described are susceptible to the development of operational definitions for research purposes and to specific testing in research design which evaluates whether families of chronic pain patients do have specific characteristics as compared with control groups. One recent study on asthmatic children failed to confirm these characteristics as specific for psychosomatic families in general, but another study of adult psychosomatic patients, the majority with chronic pain syndrome, supported the characteristics of enmeshment or social isolation and found some support for poor problem solving (16, 17).

In their study, Mohamed et al. (13) observed that families of chronic pain patients demonstrate the inability to experience and express a fantasy, private cognition or feelings and introduced the concept of "significant other specificity." These concepts suggest that certain physical complaints in the patients are unconsciously reinforced or rewarded by the spouses because of their own family problems. They found some specific evidence for this concept in that depressed patients complaining of pain had significantly more evidence of pain problems in their spouses, pain problems in the families of their spouses and a consistency of pain locations between patients and their spouse and between patients and their spouses' families than did a group of depressed patients without pain. Further, this study also provided some supportive evidence for the concept of "sick role homeostasis." In families where marital roles are dysfunctional and noncomplementary, the "sick" role may provide the family system with homeostasis, and pain takes the role of a "scapegoat." This would then provide surprising stability to a previously unstable relationship.

In summary, therefore, there is some research evidence for the role of family dynamics as precipitating and perpetuating variables in most chronic pain syndromes. Although this evidence is limited in amount, these concepts have led to treatments with a family system perspective, leading to better treatment outcomes.

THE ROLE OF MARITAL MALADJUSTMENT

Perhaps the most dramatic finding associated with chronic pain is the clear and frequently reproduced finding that marital maladjustment is a clear correlate of chronic pain. Gidro-Frank and Gordon (4), in a study of women with chronic pain, observed that the frustrating life situations centered around the marital relationships. "They felt unable to change and were dissatisfied. They had hoped to gratify excessive needs for dependence and became disturbed when faced with responsibility that marriage imposed, helpless rage towards their husbands, with depression and anxiety found by both the interviewers and the psychological tests." A second study, by Gidro-Frank and Taylor (5), revealed marked ambivalence toward their marriages, dysmenorrhea, less pleasure in orgasm and difficulty in pregnancy in a group of patients with chronic pelvic pain.

Merskey and Spear (11) demonstrated that patients with chronic pain had a 96% marriage rate, higher than the general population. They also found that sexual adjustment was poor, with impotence, frigidity and coitus interruptus. They suggest that the pain-prone patients as conceptualized by Engel (2) show a great deal of resentment in the marital situation.

Kreitman et al. (8) in 1965 in a study of patients with hypochondriasis, many of whom had chronic pain, found that their chronic pain illnesses were like those of the patients' mothers and that they had poor marital and sexual adjustment.

Recently in two separate studies, the correlation of marital maladjustment with chronic pain has been demonstrated experimentally. Mohamed et al. (13) studied patients and their spouses completing the Lock-Wallace marital adjustment scales. These authors demonstrated that depressed patients with chronic pain showed increased marital maladjustment to a highly significant degree compared with depressed patients without pain.

In summary, therefore, we have clinical and supportive research evidence suggesting that marital maladjustment is a clear correlate of chronic pain in adults and may be a perpetuating factor in the failure of these patients to respond to traditional medical, surgical or anesthetic interventions. It follows that in the assessment of patients with chronic pain syndromes, marital evaluation should be included.

Treatment

The specific role of marital counseling and/or family therapy in adults with a chronic pain syndrome is described in detail in Chapter 11. Suffice it to say that Waring et al. have used a specific form of marital and family counseling, called cognitive family therapy, with success in management of chronic pain syndromes.

Other objective trials using control groups and reliable and valid outcome criteria have demonstrated the usefulness of family oriented treatment in the chronic pain syndrome (6, 7, 9).

Waring et al. have suggested that physicians responsible for pain clinics in which the types of chronic pain syndromes we have described are being evaluated and treated could benefit from use of the General Health Questionnaire and the Lock-Wallace Marital Adjustment Scale as screening instruments, with referral of those cases with nonpsychotic emotional illness and marital maladjustment for psychiatric evaluation and treatment.

In conclusion, it has been demonstrated that chronic pain patients with marital maladjustment may not improve with traditional medical management but require, in addition, marital counseling and/or family therapy.

Acknowledgments

We wish to thank Dr. H. Merskey and Dr. E. Waring for their assistance and interest in the preparation of this chapter.

REFERENCES

1. APLEY, J. *The Child with Abdominal Pains.* Blackwell, Oxford, 1975.
2. ENGEL, W. L. Psychogenic pain and the pain prone patient. *Am. J. Med., 26:* 899–918, 1959.
3. FORDYCE, W. E. *Behavioural Methods for Chronic Pain and Illness.* C. V. Mosby, St. Louis, 1976.
4. GIDRO-FRANK, L., AND GORDON, T. Reproductive performance of women with pelvic pain of long duration. *J. Fertil. Steril., 7:* 440–447, 1956.
5. GIDRO-FRANK, L., AND TAYLOR, H. C. Pelvic pain and the female identity. *Am. J. Obstet. Gynecol., 79:* 1184–1202, 1960.
6. HUDGENS, A. J. Family oriented treatment of chronic pain. *J. Marit. Fam. Ther.,* October 1979, pp. 67–78.
7. KHATAMI, M., AND RUSH, J. A pilot study of the treatment of outpatients with chronic pain: Symptom control, stimulus control and social system intervention. *Pain 5:* 163–172, 1978.
8. KREITMAN, N., SAINSBURY, P., PEARCE, K., AND COSTAIN, W. P. Hypochondriasis and depression in out-patients at a general hospital. *Br. J. Psychiatry III:* 607–615, 1965.
9. LIEBMAN, R., HONIG, P., AND BERGER, H. An integrated treatment program for psychogenic pain. *Fam. Process, 15:* 397–405, 1976.
10. MERSKEY, H. The characteristics of persistent pain in psychological illness. *J. Psychosom. Res., 9:* 291–298, 1965.
11. MERSKEY, H., AND SPEAR, F. *Pain: Psychological and Psychiatric Aspects.* Ballière, Tindall and Cassell, London, 1967.
12. MINUCHIN, S. The use of an ecological framework in child psychiatry. In *The Child and His Family,* edited by E. J. Anthony, and C. Koupernik. Wiley, New York, 1970.
13. MOHAMED, S. N., WEISZ, G. M., AND WARING, E. M. The relationship of chronic pain to depression, marital adjustment and family dynamics. *Pain 5:* 285–292, 1978.
14. STERNBACH, R. A. *Pain Patients: Traits and Treatment.* Academic Press, New York, 1974.
15. WARING, E. M. The role of the family in symptom selection and perpetuation in psychosomatic illness. *J. Psychother. Psychosom., 28:* 253–259, 1977.
16. WARING, E. M., MOHAMED, S. N., BOYD, D. B., AND WEISZ, G. Chronic Pain and The Family. A Review Presented at the Second World Congress of the International Association for the Study of Pain, Montreal, Canada, August 1978.
17. WARING, E. M., AND RUSSELL, L. Psychosomatic Illness, Marital Maladjustment and Intimacy. Presented at the Academy of Psychosomatic Medicine, San Francisco, 1979.
18. WARNES, H. The problem of masked depression in a clinical perspective. *Psychiatr. J. Univ. Ottawa, 2:* 37–43, 1977.

11

Conjoint Marital and Family Therapy

E. M. WARING, M.D.

Chronic pain can produce suffering in the spouse and family of the patient. The chronic pain patient becomes depressed due to loss of health, loss of self-esteem, loss of income, and loss of the capacity to fill previous roles as spouse and family member. These losses also profoundly affect the patient's spouse and family. Depression, often more severe than that experienced by the chronic pain patient, is frequently found in the spouse and/or children. Thus, chronic pain can have a detrimental effect on previously well-adjusted marriages and adequately functioning families.

The reaction to chronic pain described above is understandable to professionals and families alike. Not so easily accepted is evidence that marital maladjustment and family dysfunction can play an important role in the selection of chronic pain as a symptom (22). Marital maladjustment may perpetuate chronic pain problems as do traits of a spouse such as hypochondriasis and hysteria as measured on the MMPI in at least a significant proportion of chronic pain patients (14, 18).

Clinical reports describing the use of marital counseling or conjoint family therapy in chronic pain patients will be briefly reviewed (8, 11, 12, 26). The question of whether a specific form of marital or family counseling is effective in the treatment of specific types of chronic pain patients remains to be determined.

This chapter will present a point of view regarding the importance of marital and family assessment as part of the comprehensive evaluation of all patients with chronic physical symptoms of obscure etiology and particularly chronic pain patients (1, 23). Clinical illustrations of the pragmatic value of marital and family assessment in the initial evaluation of chronic pain patients will be presented.

Three specific types of marital and family therapy which have been described in the treatment of chronic pain patients will be presented: 1) the pioneering work of Minuchin (13) and Chelune (4) using structural family therapy in the treatment of children who present with abdominal pain of obscure etiology; 2) the treatment of adult patients with "chronic pain of obscure etiology," using cognitive family therapy (19, 27); and 3) operant conditioning models to change the behavior of spouses and family members in response to chronic pain behaviors (4–6).

Finally, I will discuss the role that marital and family conjoint interviews can play in all chronic pain patients 1) to facilitate ventilation of depression, 2) to provide education which facilitates treatment adherence, and 3) to identify specific areas of marital maladjustment or family dysfunction.

Marital and/or Family Assessment

The adult patient with "chronic pain of obscure etiology" is almost invariably married or has been married (15). The chronic pain problems may have contributed to separation and/or divorce. The first major problem is arranging for a spouse and/or family to attend an assessment interview.

The pain clinic has a definite advantage since patients agree to certain conditions such as marital assessment in order to participate in the program. In the more general clinical situation where pain patients are referred randomly, the participation of the spouse or family in an assessment interview is more difficult to obtain.

I have found these general points useful in obtaining a spouse's coopera- tion. The first is to diminish the patient's pain and suffering by whatever means is effective. A patient who has received benefit from treatment (whether it be analgesics, antidepressants, biofeedback or hypnosis, to give only a few examples) will be a much more cooperative ally in obtaining the spouse's consent to participate in an assessment. Second, wherever possible, the initial treatment of a chronic pain patient should be done in the inpatient hospital setting. Spouses and families will invariably visit, allowing an opportunity to meet them and present to them the importance of a marital and/or family assessment. Finally, I tell the spouse that in my experience all spouses suffer with the chronic pain of the identified patient and that discussion of this suffering may lead to specific interventions which can improve the patient's clinical condition.

It is important to remember that in the minds of your patients and their spouses the idea that a marital relationship can have an influence on a disease or an illness is foreign and difficult for them to accept. It is a difficult idea even for the medical profession to accept! Thus, you must be willing to spend considerable time, and use clinical examples, explaining how marital assessments have led to clinical improvement in your patients.

Finally, it must also be remembered that the initial marital assessment must be a *positive* experience for both spouses if you realistically expect to have the opportunity to see them both again or to intervene positively in the marital interaction.

One of the ways of making this initial marital assessment a positive experience is to acknowledge the universal phenomenon of depression in the spouse of the chronic pain patient and allow ventilation of feelings of hopelessness and helplessness. In most assessments it is also easy to acknowledge the fact that the spouse must have experienced some frustration toward the patient and "their pain" which has gone unexpressed. Most couples will be able to acknowledge this anger on both sides which has gone unexpressed because of either guilt in expressing anger toward someone who is suffering or because of fears that anger will make the situation worse. Obviously, if the spouse denies such hostility, badgering them or insinuating that they are lying or uncooperative will lead to a negative experience.

In the initial assessment, in addition to encouraging ventilation of the depression and anger which is invariably present, I also spend considerable time in allowing the spouse expression of feelings, thoughts and expectations about being called in for a joint interview. Physicians often expect that the spouse's response will be hostile. In fact, most spouses express some relief that they have finally been brought into the treatment program. Obviously, a minority of spouses will refuse to participate in a martial interview, in which case I telephone and speak to them as described above or write a personal letter if telephoning is impossible. I also spend a good portion of the initial interview in educating both patient and spouse regarding the use of medications, such as analgesics, antidepressants, or major tranquilizers, to provide pain relief. I discuss the medical consultants who will be called in to evaluate the patient and explain ward routines, psychological testing, or other specialized modalities of treatment which may be indicated in any specific case, such as behavior modification, group therapy, or transcutaneous stimulation, to give only a few examples.

After this initial period of ventilation of attitudes, feelings, expectations, and patient education, the couple are usually in a much more receptive mood for a comprehensive marital assessment interview. Space will not allow documentation of all the areas assessed in such an interview, but suffice it to say I do a complete history of the marriage, including how the couple met, dating, courtship, engagement, honeymoon, and a chronological history of their marriage and also of their parents' marriages (19, 27).

The following areas are particularly relevant in marital assessment related to chronic pain. A history of both the patient's and the spouse's experiences with pain since childhood and the patterns of response to pain in both of their families is elicited. The family histories of pain problems and their cognitive and emotional impact on the patient and spouse are explored. The original onset of the pain problems is explored in some detail.

Specifically, I explore what the patient thought was wrong when he first experienced the pain, how this made him feel, who he first told about the pain, and what the spouse initially thought was wrong and thought should be done about the pain. Obviously, the areas of marital function which are most severely affected by chronic pain are employment, sexuality, and leisure activities, and these are explored in some depth. The *spouse's* expectations, feelings, and knowledge about the patient's physician and treatment are crucial in the marital assessment. Financial compensation to the couple as a result of disability from chronic pain as well as its meaning to them must be thoroughly explored.

The following are some clinical vignettes of initial marital assessment interviews with couples where one spouse suffers from "chronic pain of obscure etiology." These vignettes will add some relevance and meaning to the above description of the interview process. I believe they demonstrate the clinical efficacy of such interviews in terms of specific interventions which can result in relief of suffering after even a single assessment interview. Increased knowledge of marital and family factors which may be perpetuating the chronic pain problem may lead to further specific interventions to alter these perpetuating variables. Conversely, an opportunity for the treating physician to recognize factors perpetuating the chronic pain problem which either the patient, spouse, or family is unprepared to change or to acknowledge may relieve the physician of the emotional burden of attempting to cure a pain complaint which is, in effect, untreatable.

Case 1

A 44-year-old woman was referred from a gynecologist because of chronic persistent pain, demands for unnecessary surgery, and concomitant drug abuse. In her mid-twenties, the lady had had several D. & C.s for dysmenorrhea, eventually leading to a hysterectomy because of persistent, vague, crampy abdominal pain. The pain persisted, resulting a few years later in the removal of her ovaries and tubes, followed by two laparotomies for adhesions, with no specific pathology found during these operative procedures.

After some clinical improvement on antidepressants, major tranquilizers, and analgesics, a marital assessment was conducted. Her husband was extremely hostile during the initial parts of the interview. He threatened to sue the gynecologist involved unless two investigative and operative procedures which he had read about in medical journals were conducted and to withdraw his wife from the hospital and have her admitted to a famous out-of-town clinic.

The children, ages 16, 14, and 10, were clearly embarrassed and tearful regarding their father's display. Marital assessment revealed that he had always experienced morbid jealousy toward his wife during courtship and marriage. He believed that his wife would be unfaithful to him if given any opportunity. A subsequent individual interview with the husband revealed a delusional system that his wife's fidelity could only be ensured by removal of her reproductive organs. A subsequent joint interview with husband and wife explored the origins of his morbid jealousy and allowed ventilation of his wife's suffering from his unfounded accusations over the course of their marriage. The pain complaints and demands for medications ceased after the second interview. The husband was placed on a small dose of a major tranquilizer.

Although this case is a dramatic one, the contribution of the husband's beliefs, both about disease and appropriate medical treatment, to the patient's complaints of pain is not as unusual as one might believe.

Case 2

A 45-year-old man was admitted to a chronic pain clinic for treatment of low back pain persisting since a back injury many years previously.

Marital assessment revealed that at the time of the accident his wife had been furious regarding what she believed to be neglect by her husband's supervisors. She believed they caused the mishap, and their failure to inform her of the accident for several days after the event made her even more resentful.

During the interview she demonstrated hopelessness and helplessness, depressed mood, disorder of appetite and sleeping, and a conviction that no form of interview would result in a cure of her husband's chronic pain problem.

Ventilation of the wife's suffering, specific treatment with antidepressants, and education that the goals of the clinic's program was not a "cure" but "rehabilitation" led to a marked clinical improvement in the index patient's symptomatology.

Case 3

This patient was a 60-year-old woman who was brought to the psychiatry floor dramatically moaning with pain due to a postmastectomy neuralgia. The pain she complained of was in fact more likely the pain associated with myocardial infarction. A family assessment quickly led her daughter to disclose that the patient's mother had recently died of myocardial infarction and that the patient had nursed her mother through her final days. Her husband, a stoical farmer who had been unsympathetic to her complaining, became more attentive in response to his daughter's theory that her mother was, in fact, experiencing a grief reaction and denying the death of her mother by retaining a pain similar to her mother's pain. The patient became cognizant of the relationship of her pain to the death of her mother and, although the pain persisted, the patient through individual psychotherapy sessions required no further hospitalizations, surgery or analgesic medication.

Case 4

The patient was admitted to a psychiatric unit with atypical facial pain and symptoms of depression. Marital assessment revealed an affectionless marriage in which the patient's pain and interactions with physicians had become the major focus of attention of the couple. The patient refused to accept that her marriage was unfulfilling and discharged herself against medical advice.

Six months later at a chance encounter with the patient in another hospital, she said that her depression had improved and her pain had diminished. She related that she attributed his improvement to her new psychiatrist's using an MAO inhibitor antidepressant and was critical of my use of antidepressant medication of the tricyclic variety. In passing, she commented that she also had obtained a separation several months previously.

Case 5

The patient was a 35-year-old wife of a minister, who had recurrent episodes of paresis of the lower limbs accompanied by low back pain. Frequent hospitalizations had occurred with equivocal findings on investigations and with no clinical improvement having occurred. A marital assessment revealed that the wife had always resented her social role as a minister's wife. She admitted that she had feigned paresis and back pain in order to avoid social responsibility. She had avoided facing up to this behavior which she felt was shameful. The husband, in turn, revealed that he had long been convinced that she was faking but did not wish to confront her. Sessions of marital counseling focusing on the lack of trust in their relationship resulted in improved marital adjustment.

Case 6

The patient was a 60-year-old woman suffering from a polymyositis, who had chronic and persistent pain related to both muscles and joints as part of the disease process. More recently, a bilateral hip replacement continued to affect her mobility and increased her pain. She was referred because of abuse of narcotic analgesics. The patient revealed a chronic life-style of suffering and painful personal relationships, including the failure of her first marriage because of her husband's excessive drinking and physical abuse. A second marriage had resulted in their living in almost total isolation from one another. Her husband would not return home for 2 or 3 days at a time and she was trapped in her home because of her disability and inability to travel around. Marital assessment was arranged, but on two separate occasions her husband refused to come for assessment. The patient was discharged, having been withdrawn from addictive narcotic medication, but clinically unimproved although depressive symptoms were less. The referring physician was informed of the ongoing unsatisfactory marital situation which the patient was unable or reluctant to change.

In my experience, these clinical vignettes demonstrate the most common sources of marital maladjustment which perpetuate chronic pain problems. A spouse's specific psychopathology, such as a paranoid illness, depression, or active collusion with the sick role of the spouse, may perpetuate chronic physical symptoms of obscure etiology and mask serious marital maladjustment (22). The clinical vignettes also represent my experience regarding the usefulness of marital assessment in the management of chronic pain problems. The marital assessments described led to a specific, helpful intervention in 4 of the 6 cases, including major tranquilizers for the spouse of the first patient, antidepressants for the spouse of the second patient, individual psychotherapy for the patient in the third case, and marital counseling for the fifth patient. In the other 2 cases, either the spouse refused to accept a specific intervention which might have been helpful or refused to participate in the interview. As a result of the marital assessments described, improvement occurred in 4 of the 6 cases which had been referred as medical model treatment failures; in those cases in which a specific intervention could not be implemented to improve the clinical situation, a greater understanding of perpetuating factors seems to relieve some of the pressure on both patient and physician to expect or demand a cure. These cases represent my general clinical experience that a specific helpful intervention is possible in about two thirds of patients with chronic pain of obscure etiology.

Specific Conjoint Marital Therapy and Family Therapy in Chronic Pain Patients

OPERANT CONDITIONING TECHNIQUES

Liberman (11) described the use of an operant model for family therapy in the treatment of a patient with migraine in 1970. The interested reader will find a theoretical discussion of the operant model in the work of Fordyce (5).

Hudgens (8) reported her experience in using an integrated systems theory and learning theory in family oriented treatment. The general goals of the treatment program included family assessment with the plan of 1) increasing family interactions around issues other than pain, 2) improving family relationships, 3) regaining occupational roles, 4) eliminating the use of prescription pain medication, 5) increasing tolerance with selected exercise, and 6) reducing use of the health care system.

Each family had at least one close "significant other," usually the spouse of the patient, who came into the hospital two to three times a week for an hour to work with the social worker in "retraining" to ignore pain-related behavior and to reinforce health-related behavior of the patient. Later in this program, joint interviews with the patient and the spouse and then with the entire family served to examine and to treat problems such as maintaining well behaviors in the transition to the home environment.

Hudgens reported favorably on the effectiveness of this family oriented treatment utilizing specific training of the spouse in operant conditioning techniques. She suggested that a strong support system within the family is a major predictor of treatment outcome. Unfortunately, the willingness of the spouse or "significant other" to modify his or her behavior toward the patient was one criterion used for acceptance to the treatment program. They did note, however, that in the eight families in their study where the family did not modify their behavior half the patients did not succeed in maintaining treatment gains 6 months or more after the program was completed.

In summary, specific forms of marital counseling which teach the spouse to reinforce "well behaviors" in the spouse are a potentially effective technique in the treatment of some forms of medical illness, including chronic pain (8).

STRUCTURAL FAMILY THERAPY IN THE TREATMENT OF CHILDREN

Minuchin (13) described the use of structural family therapy in an integrated treatment program for children with a variety of psychosomatic illnesses including diabetes, anorexia nervosa, intractable asthma, and chronic pain. There are three general assumptions in structural family therapy: 1) The individual must be considered in terms of his membership in a number of interacting systems, and in one of these the therapist is also a member. Each system inherently tends toward homeostasis, but events may occur to alter this homeostasis in a favorable or unfavorable way. 2) Changes in behavior of a system are accompanied by change in behavior of individual members and changes in internal events in the cognitive and affective spheres. 3) The therapist enters the system with the family and is able to introduce stimulus for transactional change. Once this change has occurred in a more adaptive direction, the family, by using its own tendency toward stability and homeostasis, maintains the change.

This general approach includes concepts of roles and the complementarity of roles, patterns of communication, the ecology of the systems and subsystems, and the concept of homeostasis. As a method it has four particular characteristics which distinguish it from the traditional psychotherapies. 1) The emphasis is on the "here and now"; 2) there is emphasis on observed transactions rather than on introspection; 3) there is dependency on interactive descriptions rather than on attempting causal explanations of individual action; and 4) the style of the therapist is pragmatic, with an active interventive manner.

It has been a part of their interdisciplinary research program to identify the elements of family structure and functioning that are related to the development and reinforcement of psychosomatic symptoms in children. Almost all of these children were seriously ill at the time of referral. All the pain cases reported were diagnosed as "psychosomatic" and referred for family therapy upon the basis of independent pediatric criteria rather than upon psychiatric evaluation. Families were referred to the study group and for family therapy by the pediatricians, and they were free to receive treatment without participating in the study. Pediatricians and family therapists worked in close collaboration throughout the treatment period. The results, although lacking a control group and including other forms of behavioral treatment, have been highly encouraging. Dramatic improvement or remission of the psychosomatic symptoms has been achieved in most of these cases. Minuchin believes that the effectiveness of the therapeutic procedures can be traced to the use of the "open systems model" of psychosomatic illness and the development of therapeutic strategies based on this model. This conceptualization directs the family therapist's attention toward the context in which the psychosomatic event is initiated and maintained.

Minuchin (13) has also identified some characteristics of families with a psychosomatically disturbed child, including 1) "enmeshment," characterized by an excessive degree of responsiveness and involvement in each other's "ill behavior"; 2) "overprotectiveness," an excessive degree of concern for each other's welfare; 3) "rigidity," a commitment to maintaining the status quo; and 4) lack of conflict resolution.

MARITAL THERAPY

Descriptions of the use of marital therapy or counseling in the treatment of chronic pain patients are frequent (26). However, recent studies have demonstrated that patients with "chronic physical symptoms of obscure etiology," including chronic pain patients, have superficially adjusted marriages which mask deficiencies in interpersonal intimacy (15, 24, 28).

Marriages in which one spouse has chronic pain are frequently observed to lack intimacy. In a series of papers, intimacy has been operationally defined as one of three interpersonal dimensions which describe the quality of a marriage (25, 29). Intimacy is seen as comprising the following eight facets: 1) conflict resolution—the ease with which differences of opinions are resolved; 2) affection—the degree to which feelings of emotional closeness are expressed by the couple; 3) cohesion—a commitment to the marriage; 4) sexuality—the degree to which sexual needs are communicated and fulfilled; 5) identity—the couple's lack of self-confidence and self-esteem; 6) compatibility—the degree to which the couple is able to work and play together comfortably; 7) autonomy—the couple's degree of positive connectedness to family and friends; and 8) expressiveness—the degree to which thoughts, beliefs, attitudes and feelings are communicated within the marriage. Other operational definitions of intimacy are also available (17).

The marriages of patients with chronic pain often have one spouse who does not wish to discuss personal matters; the couples do not share feelings or engage in cognitive self-disclosure and there is a lack of affection and cohesion (20, 24, 28).

Cognitive family therapy is a technique which facilitates marital intimacy through cognitive self-disclosure. The specific technique and its effectiveness are described elsewhere (19, 27).

Jourard (9) initiated a systematic study of the phenomenon of self-disclosure which he believed was a "symptom of health" and "a means to interpersonal effectiveness." Fromm (6) discovered that self-disclosure could decrease the phenomenological distance between self and others. Chelune (4) defined self-disclosure as a process of making ourselves known to others by verbally revealing interpersonal information. Grinker (7) originally recognized that cognitive self-disclosure may be a primary determinant of a couple's level of intimacy. Brown and Harris (2) refer to "a close, confiding relationship" as a factor affecting vulnerability to depression in women under adverse circumstances, suggesting an awareness of the relationship of intimacy to self-disclosure. Murstein (16) has developed a stimulus-value interaction model to explain marital choice. He suggests that the major problem in courtship in America is that after the unconscious and conscious stimulus choice of partner, a failure to develop self-disclosure attitudes, values, and beliefs results in a lack of cognitive information which could allow marital choices when conflicting values prevent compatibility.

First, let us return to our operational definition of intimacy. Self-disclosure is seen as an important component of the "compatibility," "identity," and "expressiveness" dimensions which influence the level of marital intimacy. Thus, the quality and quantity of self-disclosure are viewed as two of several factors which can influence a couple's level of intimacy.

Jourard (9) demonstrated that personal disclosures occurred most consistently in the marital relationship. Waterman (30) reviewed studies which illustrated a positive relationship between the amount of self-disclosure and marital adjustment. Self-disclosure is facilitated when the material disclosed is perceived as appropriate and the listener is perceived as nurturant and supportive and also willing to disclose in a reciprocal pattern.

Self-disclosure can be classified as: 1) expression of emotion; 2) expression of need; 3) expression of thought, beliefs, attitudes and fantasy; and 4) self-awareness. The latter two are defined here as cognitive self-disclosure. Levinger and Senn (10) have demonstrated that there is more disclosure of negative feelings in unhappy couples. Finally, the longer an individual speaks on topics regarding the self, the more intimate the disclosures become. Sullivan (21) was the first to suggest the therapeutic value of self-disclosure. Burke et al. (3) suggest that self-disclosure can be facilitated through training or psychotherapy.

In summary, cognitive self-disclosure refers to the process of making ourselves known to others by verbally revealing personal thoughts, attitudes, beliefs and fantasy as well as developing self-awareness. A specific technique to facilitate intimacy through providing a structured exposure of a couple to self-disclosure cognitive material about their relationship, their marital choice and their parents' level of marital intimacy has been developed (19, 27). This technique, described below, is referred to as cognitive family therapy and is based on the assumption that facilitating cognitive self-disclosure will increase a couple's level of intimacy, resulting in a decrease in nonpsychotic emotional illness, including chronic pain of obscure etiology (19, 27).

The technique deliberately focuses on patterns of "thought," analyzing in detail attributions and assumptions in the family context. The therapist takes pains to facilitate self-disclosure of members until these attributions and assumptions begin to come to the fore. The approach makes the assumption that there are a number of ways of thinking which accompany dysfunctional individual and conjoint behavior: 1) arbitrary and often unfounded assumptions often play a great role in determining how things are perceived and acted upon; 2) unwarranted linkages are made between bits of data in a family—for example, a woman thinks about how she was abandoned by a former spouse, thinks about her currently unsatisfactory sexual relationship, thinks about her husband's frequent absences, and links these to conclude that her husband is having an affair because she is sexually inadequate; 3) their habits of catastrophising; and 4) generalizing, which affects the perception of "what the difficulty is." The overall approach assumes that self-disclosure is an important determinant of intimacy—it is the event in the black box that the behaviorists avoid talking about—and is an important avenue for induction of behavioral change.

CLINICAL ILLUSTRATIONS OF COGNITIVE FAMILY THERAPY

The following 2 case illustrations give a clinical picture of the use of this specific form of conjoint marital/family therapy in selected cases.

Case 1

A 43-year-old married woman who was a virtual invalid with complaints of rheumatoid arthritis was admitted for rehabilitation. Through multiple prescriptions she had been using a preparation containing acetylsalicyclic acid (ASA), codeine and phenobarbital. Her program included stepwise reductions in the abused substances with temporary addition of amitriptyline and haloperidol. Individual and group psychotherapies allowed her to express her frustration regarding her husband's habitual absences from home and her concern that he may be having an affair. This husband failed to show for two scheduled conjoint marital sessions, and when the patient was finally discharged she was more physically active, less depressed, and consuming only about one fourth of the initial dose of analgesics.

At 1 week follow-up, the husband had brought her for her appointment and was now quite willing to participate in his wife's follow-up interview. The therapist began by asking the patient to disclose her thoughts regarding her improvement; she attributed it to being away from the home where her family did practically everything for her, to conversations with others (feeling not alone in her problem), to the antidepressants and tranquilizers she had been given, and to the fact that since her discharge her husband was now spending more time with her. When her husband was asked to disclose his thoughts, he attributed the improvement to the reduction in her invalidism and in medication abuse; they both volunteered that in the past the only thing they had shared easily was their irritation.

A detailed family background was obtained from each. She spoke of her family and her losses. Recalling that her parents had never argued, she attributed this to their "good relationship" but admitted that there had been little discussion of problems or sexual issues. In her first marriage she had been abandoned by her spouse, who had left her for a woman with more money and greater sexual interest.

He recalled being the youngest of six brothers. He was only 5 when his father had died, and his mother had essentially raised the family by herself. Sexuality was not discussed in his family either and his first marriage also ended when his wife left him.

This couple met when they were both lonely and got married. After she developed phlebitis and rheumatoid arthritis, neither had the confidence for open discussion of sexual adjustment or their mutual fears of illness and disability. She was able to learn that her parents' model of never having any arguments could be attributed to the fact that they never talked about their relationship in any way, and that this accounted for her reluctance to share her concerns and lack of knowledge about sexuality with her first and second husbands. He saw that the loss of his father was a major motivation in choice of wife, looking for a family, and could see the course of his disillusionment when he had to give up his masculine self-image which he developed in a practically all male household. She was able to disclose that her chronic invalidism and pain was bringing solicitous attention from him and was able to confide her fear regarding lack of interest in sex and her fear that her disability would lead to being abandoned again. The result was that the couple had a better understanding of each other and were able to maintain an improved marital adjustment.

In this vignette, presumably the key to engagement of the husband can be attributed to the improvement in his wife and the fact that he was accompanying her to the clinic. The therapist picked the event which was apt to be concordant and dominant in both of their thought patterns at the time—the fact that improvement had occurred—and used it to open up the essentials of how they perceived their difficulties together. By encouraging self-disclosure regarding their motives for marriage and the influence of their parents' marriages and their previous marriages, background data eventually accumulated which allowed them to reconsider some of the assumptions they had made and inappropriate linkages from which they had drawn arbitrary conclusions. Her husband was neither having an affair nor planning to leave her as she supposed.

She did not have malignant intent in depriving him of his manhood by her disability. Her disability and pattern of illness behavior was not simply *her* problem but was based on their mutual defective interpretation of what was ailing. In this case the disclosure of mutually held beliefs that self-disclosure was to be avoided, because for her it was misperceived as marital adjustment and for him as nonmasculine, resulted in suffering in the role of invalid or helper as their only form of communication.

Case 2

A 34-year-old white female was admitted for treatment of recurrent backache following extensive medical workup which failed to find positive evidence for specific surgical or medical intervention.

The recent backache started about 3 weeks prior to her admission. She had insomnia and a loss of interest in sexual activity during this period.

She described herself as a lady who kept her thoughts and feelings to herself.

Her first episode of back pain was 5 years previously, after her first husband's death.

Inpatient behavioral treatment was carried on.

A marital assessment was done while the patient was in the hospital. The husband disclosed that he avoided his own thoughts and feelings and withdrew from his wife when she started to express her feelings, particularly of anger about the relationship. She experienced more backache and back pain after this initial session and acknowledged that her pain was much worse when she was withholding or thinking about her anger in the interpersonal situation.

The wife disclosed during the second interview an extensive history of surgical interventions resulting in hysterectomy and bilateral removal of both breasts due to fibrous nonmalignant nodules. She disclosed that she had also experienced low back pain during the birth of her three children from her previous marriage. She disclosed her thoughts regarding her loss of female reproductive organs through surgery saying, "God had a good reason for giving me these things, and I'm sure he has a better reason for taking them away." She disclosed that her first husband had drunk excessively and in subsequent sessions disclosed that she was aware that this was in part, at least, produced by her lack of interest in sexuality.

Her spouse said that their marriage, her second marriage, had been a good marriage for 4 years. He disclosed that he had been attracted by the fact that she had children; he had wanted to have children and, in fact, had adopted her three children now ages 16, 14, and 12.

The third cognitive family therapy session focused specifically on both partners' experiences in their own family with knowledge and attitudes regarding sexuality and more specifically their difficulties in the current relationship. They both agreed that arguments which ensued in the family were related to sexual frustration.

Sessions focused on his lack of information about sexuality in his background, shame and embarrassment about masturbation and inability to discuss his sexual needs with his wife. His sexual inexperience led him to pick a woman who already had three children and who had had mastectomies and a hysterectomy, thus he believed relieving him of anxiety regarding sexual performance. These beliefs were superficially discussed but were felt to be an area which further insight on his part might do more harm than good.

During these sessions the wife focused on her lack of trust of men and on the influence of her mother's attitude which contributed to sexual frustration in both her first and second marriages. The couple felt considerably more understanding of one another as a result of these interviews, and her pain diminished to the point where she could actively involve herself in recreation, work, and sexual intercourse; at 6 month follow-up, the patient continued to be well.

The rationale for improvement in the second case is the couple's self-disclosure of their sexual attitudes. The husband's lack of knowledge and inexperience were revealed, and his sexually demanding behavior was found to be more related to feeling left outside of the family and envy of the children than to genuine sexual desire. The self-disclosure of their compatibility in lack of libido made it easier for the wife to meet his needs for closeness in the nonsexual area and for him to respond to her without her use of the sick role.

Cognitive family therapy assumes that where chronic pain of obscure etiology is perpetuated by marital maladjustment, facilitating cognitive self-disclosure will increase intimacy, reducing the necessity for abnormal illness behavior to elicit caring from spouse and professionals. Cognitive family therapy is presented as one example of marital and/or family therapy in the treatment of chronic pain because it is the technique the author is most familiar with in clinical practice and not necessarily as the best or only approach.

Summary

Marital and family assessment is indicated in all patients with "chronic pain of obscure etiology" and will provide valuable information with facilitation of treatment programs. Studies of specific forms of family or marital therapy for chronic pain patients are preliminary and uncontrolled but are encouraging. Finally, only three specific techniques, viz., 1) operant conditioning training for the spouse, 2) cognitive family therapy and 3) structural family therapy, have been reported in the treatment of chronic pain patients. Two cases treated with cognitive family therapy are described as examples. It must be emphasized that marital and family therapy is not the only treatment for patients with chronic pain.

Further evaluation of conjoint marital and/or family therapy for patients with chronic pain is needed. It should be noted that evaluation of the effectiveness of family therapy in patients who are also participating in behavior modification, therapeutic medication, and physical treatment is difficult because of these confounding variables. A controlled research design is a prerequisite to evaluating the effectiveness of a specific form of family therapy.

Chronic pain results in suffering for patient, spouse, family and physician. Effective assessments and intervention with couples and families will diminish this suffering in the majority of cases. Specific forms of conjoint marital and/or family therapy may be helpful in patients in whom marital and/or family maladjustment contributes to the perpetuation of chronic pain.

REFERENCES

1. ALGER, I. Family therapeutic approaches to the medically ill patient. In *Psychotherapeutics in Medicine*, edited by T. B. Karasu, and R. I. Steinmuller. Grune and Stratton, New York, 1978, pp. 203–222.
2. BROWN, G. W., AND HARRIS, T. Social origins of depression: A reply. *Psychol. Med., 8:* 577–588, 1978.
3. BURKE, R. J., WEIR, T., AND DUWORDS, R. E. Type A behaviour of administrators and wives: Report of marital satisfaction and well-being. *J. Appl. Psychol., 64(1):* 57–65, 1979.
4. CHELUNE, G. J. Nature and assessment of self-disclosing behaviour. In *Advances in Psychological Assessment*, Vol. 4, edited by P. McReynolds. Jossey-Bass, San Francisco, 1978.
5. FORDYCE, W. E. *Behavioural Methods for Chronic Pain and Illness.* Mosby, St. Louis, 1976.
6. FROMM, E. *The Sane Society.* Holt, Rinehart and Winston, New York, 1955.
7. GRINKER, R. Intimacy: Definitions and distortions. In *Sex, Love and Intimacy—Whose Life Styles?* Report from Second Annual S.I.E.C.U.S. Conference, Nobember 5, 1971, New York.
8. HUDGENS, A. J. Family oriented treatment of chronic pain. *J. Marit. Fam. Ther.*, October 1979, pp. 67–78.
9. JOURARD, S. M. *The Transparent Self.* Van Nostrand Reinhold, Princeton, NJ, 1964.
10. LEVINGER, G., AND SENN, D. J. Disclosure of feelings in marriage. *Merrill Palmer Q. 13:* 237–249, 1967.
11. LIBERMAN, R. Behavioral approaches to family and couple therapy. *Am. J. Orthopsychiatry 40:* 106–118, 1970.

12. LIEBMAN, R. An integrated treatment program for psychogenic pain. *Fam. Process 15:* 397, 1976.
13. MINUCHIN, S. The use of an ecological framework in child psychiatry. In *The Child and His Family*, edited by E. J. Anthony, and C. Koupernik, Wiley, New York, 1970.
14. MOHAMED, S. N. The patient and his family. In *Chronic Pain: Psychosocial Factors in Rehabilitation*, edited by R. Roy and E. Tunks. Williams & Wilkins, Baltimore, 1982, chap. 10.
15. MOHAMED, S. N., WEISZ, G. M., AND WARING, E. M. The relationship of chronic pain to depression, marital adjustment and family dynamics. *Pain 5:* 285–292, 1978.
16. MURSTEIN, B. I. *Love, Sex, and Marriage Through the Ages.* Springer Publications, New York, 1974.
17. OLSON, D. H., AND SCHAEFER, M. T. *Diagnosing Intimacy: The PAIR Inventory.* Presented at the National Council on Family Relations Annual Conference, San Diego, 1977.
18. ROBERTS, A. H. The behavioural management of chronic pain: Long-term follow-up with comparison groups. *Pain 8:* 151–162, 1980.
19. RUSSELL, A., RUSSELL, L., AND WARING, E. M. Cognitive family therapy: A preliminary report. *Can. Psychiatr. Assoc. J. 25:* 64–67, 1980.
20. SIFNEOS, P. E. Problems of psychotherapy of patients with alixothymic characteristics and physical disease. *Psychother. Psychosom. 26(2):* 65–70, 1975.
21. SULLIVAN, H. S. *The Interpersonal Theory of Psychiatry.* Norton Press, New York, 1953.
22. WARING, E. M. The role of the family in symptom selection and perpetuation in psychosomatic illness. *Psychother. Psychosom. 28(1–4):* 253–259, 1977.
23. WARING, E. M. Psychosomatic symptoms and marital adjustment. *Psychiatr. Forum 8(2):* 9–13, 1979.
24. WARING, E. M. Marital intimacy, psychosomatic symptoms, and cognitive therapy. *Psychosomatics 21:* 595–601, 1980.
25. WARING, E. M., McELRATH, D., WEISZ, G. M., AND LEFCOE, D. Aspects of intimacy in young couples. *Psychiatry*, in press.
26. WARING, E. M., MOHAMED, S. N., BOYD, D. B., AND WEISZ, G. *Chronic Pain and the Family: A Review.* Presented at the Second World Congress of the International Association for the Study of Pain, Montreal, Canada, August 1978.
27. WARING, E. M., AND RUSSELL, L. Cognitive family therapy: An outcome study. *J. Sex Marit. Ther. 6(4):* Winter 1980.
28. WARING, E. M., AND RUSSELL, L. Family structure, marital adjustment, and intimacy in general hospital psychiatry consultation—liaison patients. *Gen. Hosp. Psychiatry 3(3):* 198–203, 1980.
29. WARING, E. M., TILLMANN, M. P., FRELICK, L., RUSSELL, L., AND WEISZ, G. Concepts of intimacy in the general population. *J. Nerv. Ment. Dis. 168(8):* 471–474, 1980.
30. WATERMAN, J. Self-disclosure and family dynamics. In *The Anatomy of Self-Disclosure*, edited by G. Chelune. Jossey-Bass, San Francisco, in press.

12

Group Therapy: A Specific Model

SUSAN BAPTISTE, Reg. O.T.
EDITH HERMAN, D.P.T., M.H.Sc.

History of Groups

The history of group therapy would require a text of its own and has been reviewed by several authors in the past two decades (Sadock in 1975 (25) and Levi-Strauss in 1963 (15), for example). A brief outline is undertaken here, with particular reference to the group approach with chronic disease processes.

The physician who initiated the use of groups as a therapeutic intervention was neither a psychiatrist nor a psychologist but an internist, Joseph Hersley Pratt, working at a Massachusetts sanatorium (25). His patients shared a common problem, a debilitating disease with poor prognosis. They were despondent about their future and experienced isolation and ostracism from the community. Pratt organized educational classes for these patients, during which he would lecture on the disease and answer their questions with honesty, always stressing the positive. (Modern practitioners might call this a "cognitive approach.")

He also encouraged patient participation by prompting them to share their concerns. In this supportive and encouraging climate, changes in patients' attitude soon became obvious. The most interesting phenomenon, however, was that the patients who benefited the most from the group meetings soon began to influence other members (a process we call "modeling") and the group as a whole responded favorably to this treatment. Many present day self-help groups, such as Alcoholics Anonymous, use precisely the same techniques with acclaimed success.

In 1919, a psychiatrist, Cody Marsh, utilized Pratt's methods with institutionalized patients, while concurrently E. W. Lazell, of the same medical discipline, also used a didactic approach to reduce fear in schizophrenic patients. Many other psychiatrists during the 1920s and 1930s selected group methods as viable treatment interventions. Adler was the major exponent of group therapy in Europe; he felt strongly about providing help to the lower classes, because his focus was on the social nature of the problems of the human condition (25, 33).

By the later 1930s, despite the fact that group therapy had not yet been labeled as a bona fide treatment methodology, many more physicians began using it and applying it to a variety of patient groups: Wender, with hospitalized nonpsychotic patients (33); Burrows and Schilder, with psychoneurotic outpatients (3, 33); and Slavson, with emotionally disturbed children and adolescents (33).

World War II increased the use of treatment groups, due to the much larger number requiring help and the necessity to meet this demand in the most economical way.

Group methods are now widely used by many disciplines. Although the methods of different group therapies vary with underlying theories, it is interesting to note that group psychotherapy itself traces its roots to a "cognitive approach."

Group Methods for Chronic Pain Patients

There has been some effort over the past years to conceptualize chronic pain not in the medical model but in a learning paradigm (9). Pain behavior may include "learned helplessness" (26) which is based on the experience of failure in the past and the perception that outcomes have little to do with one's own efforts. Being the passive recipient of often ineffective treatments only serves to perpetuate the problem and results in a "giving up" attitude (6). Since dysfunctional cognitions, emotions and behaviors are common to all chronic pain patients, this syndrome lends itself well to group methods not unlike those used by Pratt in the early part of the century.

Stressing the "here-and-now" of interactional group methods, the purpose of the group is to correct misconceptions about pain through education and to provide instructions for pain control. Inherent in the group is an opportunity for problem solving, interpersonal learning and learning by modeling. The climate of mutual support and encouragement in a diagnostically homogeneous group not only facilitates learning but also serves as a "corrective emotional experience" (33, p. 18). Moreover, verbal communication in itself has therapeutic value: it competes with negative thoughts, increases self-confidence and facilitates interpersonal learning (18). Whatever the psychological approach employed, the final goal is to replace "learned helplessness" with "learned resourcefulness" (26).

Thus, the major goal of group programs for patients with chronic pain is to augment autonomy. The patient has to assume responsibility for his rehabilitation in order to become independent. This involves a reverse learning process from the way he "learned" his pain behavior, concomitant attitudes and thinking styles. Learning, however, not only is an intellectual exercise but also involves an experiential process which requires involvement and active participation. Above all, opportunity for mastery over some aspect of the pain problem has to be provided to improve self-concept. Reconstitution of self-esteem is particularly crucial to the rehabilitation of the chronic pain patient with a history of failures, the antecedent of helplessness.

Effective Ingredients of Group Therapy for Chronic Pain

Turk and Genest (31) integrated an extensive review of literature on stress responses, laboratory studies on pain and cognitive-behavioral research; they applied it to a comparison of three different clinical group approaches to chronic pain. Despite different approaches, there are similarities in conceptualization and common elements which account for therapeutic change in patients. Fordyce's (8, 9) "behavior modification program" is based on an operant model which manipulates the consequences maintaining pain behavior (attention, rest, medication etc.). Sternbach (28) and others base their approach on transactional group strategies and social learning; patients learn to recognize each other's "pain games" and to replace them with more adaptive behavior.

Gottlieb's comprehensive rehabilitation program offers a combination of various treatment strategies (group therapy, physiotherapy, occupational therapy, biofeedback, relaxation, counseling); it is the model for most present-day pain programs. Turk and Genest (31) stated that the basic assumption underlying all approaches is that the pain experience can be altered by psychological interventions. A crucial element responsible for behavioral change in each case lies in the fact that the "successful" patient changes his conceptualization of the pain problem. All group programs, therefore, are based on a "translation" process during which the patient learns to view his problem in a different way.

Effective ingredients to produce therapeutic change are, therefore, positive expectations (indispensable for generating the necessary motivation), a change in cognition and attitude and, finally, a sense of mastery (10, 11, 13, 14).

A Specific Group Method

The following is an account of the pain control program at McMaster University Medical Centre Division which has been in operation for over 3 years and has proven to be an effective component within the rehabilitation department and as a resource to the pain clinic. The operation of the group will be discussed below. The relative success of the program can probably be attributed to a variety of different factors which may be deliberately designed within the program or may be seen to be a by-product of the program. These factors deserve some attention at this point.

EXPECTATION

Expectation for a positive outcome is recognized as one of the most important ingredients in successful psychotherapy (11). Expectation is, no doubt, the basis of the placebo response; by the same token it may account for the "negative therapeutic reaction" or the side effects of which patients often complain when they are anxious or their level of trust is low. Patients referred to a program for chronic pain often see this agency as a "court of last appeal" and they bring with them a mixture of great hopes and great fears. The mobilization of positive expectations can be one of the most important tasks in bringing about therapeutic change; in fact, it may be the key. Some of the expectations of positive outcome will come simply from the need the sufferer brings with him to finally find a solution. Some positive expectation may come by reputation or from exposure to individuals who have had a good experience in that program. Positive expectation can be deliberately engendered by an educational program by defining the objectives and realistically portraying the possible range of outcomes, based on previous experience of the program. This sort of intervention at the beginning of a program might be considered an "indoctrination" but probably is a common element in every kind of psychotherapy.

A CLIMATE OF SUPPORT

The client centered approach to psychotherapy as described by Carl Rogers includes the necessary element of "unconditional positive regard," accurate empathy and genuineness (22, 23). (The matter of positive regard and alliance is considered a sine qua non of a good therapeutic relationship even by laymen, who will often change or choose their physician or therapist simply on the basis of that criterion.)

The presence of this factor implies both that the therapist will demonstrate an attitude of encouragement and caring and that this will be more or less successfully communicated to his client or patient. The group setting of patients with similar problems may provide an additional basis for a sense of being understood. In fact, it is a frequent observation by graduates of pain control groups that what they appreciated most was the realization that they were not "alone" and that their problem could be understood by others. It follows from this that the constitution of a group for chronic pain must be conducive to such a climate. Therapists must be individually suited to dealing with the frustrations and often annoying problems associated with chronic disability and pain.

IMPARTING OF INFORMATION (UNDERSTANDING)

Man fears most what he does not know. Relevant information serves to dispel myths and misconceptions about pain; this, in turn, reduces anxiety, a powerful concomitant of pain which significantly increases its perceived severity (21, 27, 31).

In one group, 2 patients began to talk about their back pain and their understanding that they were suffering from "slipped discs." It became evident after a while that their fantasies about what "slipped discs" really meant were exaggerated and frightening—notions of a spine crumbling away, paralysis setting in and deterioration slowly working its way through the body with each new pain. When clarification was given to these patients that their discs had not really "slipped" and they understood that instead there was some degree of weakening and bulging within parts of these discs, they were noticeably less anxious.

New information provides the basis for problem solving and behavioral change. One way of looking at this process was formulated by Festinger (7). According to that notion, integrating new information which is inconsistent with presently held beliefs prompts the individual to rearrange his cognitive elements. If this new information is persuasive enough to be accepted, there may be a state of "cognitive dissonance" between this new belief and the behavior of the individual which is not congruent with this new belief. Since it is psychologically not comfortable to sustain this incongruency between belief and previous behavior, the individual may respond by altering his behavior in accordance with the new belief (34). The new behavior may now be sustained because of the reduction of dissonance and discomfort.

The imparting of information may permit a sufferer to call into question fears which themselves have posed a problem. For example, an individual with chronic pain may believe that he has no control over his pain or his life events. (This psychological trait has been called "locus of control" and certain psychological tests such as the internal/external locus of control scale (24) have been devised to describe this characteristic.)

Information provided may give a subject substantial reason to begin to act in a more assertive and adaptive way. To obtain a therapeutic effect requires a good deal of congruency between the conceptualization of the patient and the conceptualization of the therapist, since this shared opinion will form the basis of goals and focus for intervention (31).

Other very important information probably communicated in any successful therapy concerns 1) the norms that govern the therapeutic activity, 2) rules of a commitment and 3) acceptance of personal responsibility. This type of information may be conveyed covertly or overtly.

COGNITIVE RESTRUCTURING

It has been popular lately to talk in terms of a newer trend in therapy called "the cognitive psychotherapy" or "cognitive-behavioral therapy" (2, 17, 19, 20). The basic thesis is that maladaptive behaviors are often predicated on maladaptive patterns and content of thinking. There may, for example, be self-defeating attitudes or negative self-statements which have become automatic. The first step in retraining (cognitive restructuring) involves bringing to the patients's awareness and acknowledgement the existence of these "internal statements"; for example, what is he saying to himself while he is in pain? An example of such analysis is found in Table 12.1. A detailed enquiry identifies the environmental events which precipitate the problem in question; patients then learn to identify and verbalize their "internal dialogues" that are likely to occur in those situations.

As these statements are verbalized, the individual may recognize the existence of some irrational fears and beliefs; an opportunity can then be made for adopting other alternatives more apt to be successful for coping. These alternatives may simply be taught or may be learned from others who are demonstrating them. After some practice has been carried out to become comfortable with these new adaptive strategies in simulated stress situations, efforts are directed toward practicing these skills during exposure to a variety of more stressful situations that would usually result in anxiety, pain or other distress. The patients are encouraged to have more than one adaptive strategy at their disposal and to include a "fail safe" mechanism such as "I can't expect miracles!" (31).

TABLE 12.1. *Cognitive Restructuring and Self-Guidance*

Situation	Internal Statement	Revised Statement	Reinforcing Statement
Driving a car on a freeway, suddenly feeling over-whelmed by low back pain	The pain is killing me . . . It's unbearable . . . I'm trapped . . . Something terrible is going to happen . . . I can't cope	I feel panicky . . . There is no reason to panic . . . I am not trapped . . . I could always pull over, stop the car, stretch out . . . I have a choice! I can handle it a little longer . . . one step at a time	
		First, I start to breathe regularly and calmly . . .	Good! That's better
		Now, I let go of my muscle tension	That's better than last time
		I can control the level of pain	
	But I'm still in so much pain . . .	Can't expect miracles . . . I'm O.K. if I just continue	
		I won't think of pain, but rather of place in which I felt good.	It works! I'm calmer now . . .
		It's really not that bad	Pain is easing
		I've coped with worse	I'm doing splendidly
		I can do it	
		Relax some more . . .	Wait till I tell the group . . .
		Pain has definitely eased	Good! I'm in control

SYSTEMATIC DESENSITIZATION OR COUNTERCONDITIONING

Systematic desensitization or counterconditioning may be seen as an element of relaxation training, autogenic training, some hypnotic procedures, role playing and a number of other techniques that are used in various therapeutic situations. The idea is that if a response inhibitory to anxiety can be made to occur in the presence of the anxiety-evoking stimulus, it will weaken the bond between the two (32). However, it should also be mentioned that relaxation techniques for chronic pain patients are not simply employed for desensitization or for counterconditioning of anxiety but also are intended to teach the individual to discriminate internal cues for tension and other feelings. By recognizing and controlling these cues, the patient begins to experience a sense of mastery. One of the greatest problems experienced by patients with pain is the apprehension that pain will become unbearable or that they will suddenly become immobilized or helpless in the case of a new attack of pain. Education, group programs or relaxation programs for pain patients often serve to "desensitize" the patient to such apprehensions.

One patient reported an interesting incident which took place after a second road accident, this time after she had had some instruction in the pain control classes. Although she was experiencing marked pain from her original pain source, plus further new pain from injuries and reasonable fear of critical damage, she "controlled" her situation. In fact, her behavior was such that it elicited an astonished response from the ambulance attendant who could not understand how the patient could have such obvious injuries (and presumably pain) and appear to be so relaxed. She told the group that when she noted anxiety, she was able to cope effectively by employing the learned principles of relaxation and rehearsing her cognitive repertoire.

OPERANT CONDITIONING

Operant learning/conditioning principles are employed by rewarding (via praise or attention) every behavioral change in the desired direction. Literature on operant conditioning is extensive and the application to the treatment of pain has been well-known since the publication of Fordyce's work (8, 9).

A middle-aged gentleman arrived for each group session exhibiting obvious pain behavior: use of two canes, stiff posture and gait. He continually grimaced, shifted in his chair and uttered audible groans at regular intervals, all of which produced virtually no response from his fellow group members or therapists. However, he did receive commendation when he did not exhibit pain behavior for a significant period. Following this incident it was noted that he displayed less and less obvious pain behavior. He began to laugh and talk more and appeared more relaxed in posture. He eventually gave up his canes. The group responded to each of these changes with enthusiasm and he continued to improve.

Appropriate cues that signal what behavior is expected and what behavior is apt to be rewarded are important elements in behavioral change. Here one sees the importance of establishing at the very beginning of a therapeutic contract the "rules" and expectations by which group members govern themselves. Clarifying these rules serves as a guideline not only for therapists but also for group members to thereafter govern their interpersonal responses according to group norms.

"Assertiveness training" also could be seen as an aspect of operant conditioning. Deficient response repertoires and problem solving ability result in inadequate performance and inappropriate feedback from the environment. Lack of assertiveness which may reflect lack of confidence and sense of security probably have much to do with the ability to cope with stress and to solve problems. Toomey et al. (30) suggested that there was a significant correlation between refractoriness to somatic treatment (acupuncture) and measures of submissiveness and passivity. Lazarus (14) found that patients with low assertiveness had deficient repertoires to cope with stress.

One of the ways of bringing about more adaptive and assertive behaviors is by the use of "role playing." Obviously this is not the only method, but it is a very effective and easily employed technique, particularly with individuals who are having difficulties with adaptation, for example, to chronic pain.

Not infrequently, it becomes apparent during role play that repertoires of "coping" and "well-behaviors" from the past are still present but are unused because "helplessness" was "learned" by conditioned anxiety and repeated frustration due to the chronic pain problem. These healthier behaviors can be successfully resurrected during role play. Obviously too, there is an element of reward in a successful performance, even though it be "played," and learning may take place by active role playing as well as by observing.

Mrs. D., a 30-year-old housewife, had suffered back pain since an auto accident 2 years before and since then had had to forego her career as a graphic artist. In the group, she appeared depressed, complained of being irritable and "not being appreciated" at home. The fact that since her ailment her husband was frequently away confirmed her sense of failure. She was asked during one session to leave the room and reenter it a few minutes later, imagining herself "1 year later and completely pain-free." She then had to field questions of other group members who were asking her "how she did it." Initially self-conscious and faltering in her answers, she gradually changed as the group became more involved. Her answers became more assured and the ways of "how she had overcome her problem" ever more inventive, so much so that by the end of the session she stated to her surprise that she was free of pain. She was asked to repeat this "game" at home, meeting different situations with the same approach. Rather significant improvement in her adjustment resulted.

Social skills and confidence in a social situation may be improved by such learning processes, and success of new adaptive maneuvers themselves becomes reinforcing for further change.

It should be noted that the "stress inoculation" procedures described by

Meichenbaum and Turk (20) are quite analogous to the factors and maneuvers mentioned above.

MODELING

Modeling is one of the most powerful influences in group therapy. It refers to the acquisition of new forms of behavior (or thinking) by observation of the behavior and the behavioral outcomes of others (1). Craig (5) found that the impact of models on pain tolerance was even greater than the influence of personality factors, "locus of control" beliefs or direct instructions. Seeing the beneficial effect of applied coping strategies in others often may prompt an observer to examine his own strategies, reevaluate their appropriateness or even reinterpret his distorted perceptions. It should be recognized too that attitudes themselves can be modeled (4, 5), provided that the modeling is realistic and believable; enhanced when there is a similarity between the model and the observer, the modeling response can be quite pronounced and long lasting. The modeling effect of the therapists should not be ignored; it is often helpful to have a therapist in a pain group who has undergone a pain problem of some chronicity. Such therapists may serve as ideal role models. Modeling effects can also be produced by inviting successful members of previous programs to participate or speak.

The converse, a detrimental modeling effect, may occur when the group holds too large a number of individuals who are not committed to the group's goal and norms. The therapeutic effectiveness of the group may be undermined by these negative modeling effects (29).

The Pain Control Classes

In over 3 years of operation, the pain control classes, which are conducted conjointly by the Departments of Physiotherapy and Occupational Therapy, have enjoyed considerable popularity and have served both hospital and community at large as well as the pain clinic (12).

The criteria for acceptance into the program are that pain must have persisted longer than 6 months, must be refractory to conventional treatment and must be the cause of dysfunction. Patients are never accepted for psychological reasons—they must experience chronic pain.

Fourteen patients are accepted in each group, which meets twice a week for 9 weeks, each session lasting 1½ hr. Sessions include group discussions, role playing, analysis of thought processes and interactions as well as other techniques, alternating with general relaxation practice.

The results of the program on a pilot sample were reported elsewhere (13). Of 75 patients, 61% were female, 39% male. Age range was 21 to 71 years, with an average of 46 years. Seventy-three percent were married, 32% were in receipt of Workmen's Compensation Board benefits or had litigation pending and 20% were gainfully employed, with the remainder either unemployed or housewives. With regard to pain, 61% were low back sufferers,

25% had head and neck pain and the remainder presented with other sources of pain. Pain duration ranged from 6 months to 30 years, with a chronicity of 3 years being most common; 50% of chronic back pain patients had had pain for more than 5 years. Thirty-seven percent of all patients had had from one to four surgeries for their pain. At least some degree of psychological or social dysfunction or distress was noted in 87% of the patients. The majority had had psychiatric interviews and many had come for at least one marital or family interview; 54% of the patients continued to receive psychopharmacological or psychotherapeutic treatment during the several weeks of group attendance.

Evaluation of outcome was based on pain intensity at best and worst times, activity level plus perception of impairment, drug intake, level of depression and locus of control. Pretest and posttest measures on these variables were obtained using standardized instruments. The final evaluation comprised 10 categories and included also the patient's cognitive control, an attitudinal questionnaire, the patient's judgment of the program's value as well as therapists' judgment of the patient's participation and progress, and a form completed by the patient's case manager. The patient's overall improvement was determined by converting the accumulated points across 10 categories (with a maximum score of 20 points) to a percentage basis. A change of 39% or less was considered a failure.

On postprogram evaluation, 79% of the patients demonstrated improvement to various degrees, although not necessarily in the same areas. Most noticeable was the marked decrease of depression scores ($P = 0.001$) and pain perception ($P = 0.001$). The shift toward perceived internal control ($P = 0.06$) was reflected in positive attitude changes.

The fact that analgesic intake is drastically reduced for the majority of patients on admission to the pain clinic could account for the findings that decrease of medication during group attendance did not reach the level of significance. Twenty-one previously unemployed group participants returned to work within a few months after completing the program.

It is interesting to note that a change of thought patterns (or the lack of it) distinguished the "successes" from the "failures." The former were much more likely to employ cognitive strategies when coping with stress.

Group Indoctrination

As each new series begins, all of the members listen to the therapist explain that "we do not cure you—you cure yourselves; we are here to help you accomplish that goal." A commitment is required of all the members for regular attendance and compliance, for the willingness to change some personal self-defeating habits, and for taking personal responsibility for the outcome.

Group norms have to be developed. For example, in one group some group members with "terrible" back pain were allowed to lie down during the group proceedings—the result was an epidemic of similar behavior on the part of other members. Therefore, at the beginning, rules for comportment are laid out. Another rule in which all members share is that any positive change will be verbally or nonverbally given recognition.

Several sessions are devoted to providing a framework and language that will assist the patients in discussing their personal problems, while at the same time giving them a rationale that will allow them to do some problem solving toward more appropriate coping. Some time is spent with specific group discussion about the role of cognition and "self-talk" as well as discussion of the relationship of the relaxation response to a sense of self-control and pain reduction. The role of medications and the attitudes they engender of not being in personal control are also important topics of discussion. With succeeding sessions the therapists take less of a directive role, gradually facilitating active participation, discussion and expression by group members. As self-disclosure becomes more common, specific situations may be dealt with through role playing. During the 9-week course, all patients keep diaries of their mood, pain, activity and medication; this enables them to mark their progress in these areas and provides the basis for evaluation at the end of the program. The results are publicly shared and serve as further reinforcement for adaptive change.

Follow-up of these patients after discharge from the program shows that the beneficial results are long lasting and that, overall, about 80% of graduates feel that their participation in the program was worthwhile.

Summary

Group programs have proven their worth in a variety of situations. Although they tend in the minds of most people to be associated with psychiatric practice, it is instructive to note that in fact they had their earliest beginnings among patients who suffer chronic disease; it is among patients suffering chronic pain that the use of groups is now beginning to flourish. There are a number of possible group approaches from which to choose, including, for example, transactional, educational and cognitive models. No matter what particular model or technique is being employed, it is likely that there are a number of similar effective ingredients inherent in the group process. Awareness of these ingredients as well as active structuring and manipulation of them will enhance the effectiveness of the group. The particular experience of the McMaster pain control classes was discussed as a case in point of a group with a strong cognitive-behavioral orientation, stressing education and relaxation techniques.

REFERENCES

1. BANDURA, A., BLANCHARD, E. B., AND RITTER, B. Relative efficacy of desensitization and modelling approaches for inducing behavioural, affective and attitudinal changes. *J. Pers. Soc. Psychol., 13:* 173–199, 1969.

2. BECK, A. *Cognitive Therapy and the Emotional Disorders.* International Universities Press, New York, 1976.
3. BURROWS, T. The group method of analysis. *Psychoanal. Rev., 19:* 268–280, 1927.
4. CRAIG, K. D. Social modelling determinants of pain processes. *Pain 1:* 375–378, 1975.
5. CRAIG, K. D. Social modelling influences on pain. In *The Psychology of Pain*, edited by R. A. Sternbach. Raven Press, New York, 1978.
6. ENGEL, G. L. A life setting conducive to illness: The giving-up, given-up complex. *Ann. Intern. Med., 69:* 293–300, 1968.
7. FESTINGER, L. *Theory of Cognitive Dissonance.* Harper & Row, New York, 1957.
8. FORDYCE, W. E. Behavioural concepts in chronic pain and illness. In *The Behavioural Management of Anger, Depression and Pain*, edited by P. O. Davidson. Bruner/Mazel, New York, 1976, pp. 147–187.
9. FORDYCE, W. E. Learning processes in pain. In *The Psychology of Pain*, edited by R. A. Sternbach. Raven Press, New York, 1978, pp. 49–72.
10. FRANK, J. D. *Persuasion and Healing: A Comparative Study of Psychotherapy.* Johns Hopkins University Press, Baltimore, 1973.
11. FRANK, J. D., ET AL. *Effective Ingredients of Successful Psychotherapy.* Bruner/Mazel, New York, 1978.
12. HERMAN, E., AND BAPTISTE, S. E. Pain control mastery through group experience. Submitted and accepted for publication, J. Kane, 1980.
13. HOEHN-SARIC, R. Emotional arousal, attitude change and psychotherapy. In *Effective Ingredients of Successful Psychotherapy*, edited by J. D. Frank. Bruner/Mazel, New York, 1978.
14. LAZARUS, R. S. A cognitive analysis of biofeedback control. In *Biofeedback: Theory and Research*, edited by G. E. Schwartz, and J. Beatty. Academic Press, New York, 1977, pp. 67–87.
15. LEVI-STRAUSS, C. *Structural Anthropology.* Basic Books, New York, 1963, pp. 167–185.
16. LIBERMAN, B. L. The role of mastery in psychotherapy: Maintenance of improvement and prescriptive change. In *Effective Ingredients of Successful Psychotherapy*, edited by J. D. Frank. Bruner/Mazel, New York, 1978, pp. 35–72.
17. MAHONEY, M. J. *Cognition and Behaviour Modification.* Ballinger, Cambridge, MA, 1974.
18. McLEAN, P. Therapeutic decision-making in the behavioural treatment of depression. In *The Behavioural Management of Anger, Depression and Pain*, edited by P. O. Davidson. Bruner/Mazel, New York, 1976, pp. 54–90.
19. MEICHENBAUM, D. *Cognitive Behaviour Modification: An Integrative Approach.* Plenum Press, New York, 1977.
20. MEICHENBAUM, D., AND TURK, D. The cognitive-behavioural management of anxiety, anger and pain. In *The Behavioural Management of Anger, Depression and Pain*, edited by P. O. Davidson. Bruner/Mazel, New York, 1976, pp. 1–34.
21. MELZACK, R. *The Puzzle of Pain.* Penguin Books, Harmondsworth, England, 1973.
22. ROGERS, C. The necessary and sufficient conditions of therapeutic personality change. J. Consult, Psychol., *21:* 95–103, 1957.
23. ROGERS, C. A theory of therapy, personality and interpersonal relationships. In *Psychology: A Study of a Science, Vol. 3*, edited by S. Koch. McGraw-Hill, New York, 1959, pp. 184–256.
24. ROTTER, J. B. Generalized expectations for internal versus external control of reinforcement. *Psychol. Monogr., 80:* 609, 1966.
25. SADOCK, B. J. Group psychotherapy. In *Comprehensive Textbook of Psychiatry*, edited by A. Freedman, H. I. Kapland, and B. J. Sadock. Williams & Wilkins, Baltimore, 1975.
26. SELIGMAN, M. E. P. *Helplessness.* W. H. Freeman, San Francisco, 1975.
27. STERNBACH, R. A. *Pain Patients: Traits and Treatment.* Academic Press, New York, 1974.

28. STERNBACH, R. A. (Ed.) *The Psychology of Pain.* Raven Press, New York, 1978.
29. SWANSON, D. W., SWENSON, W. M., MARUTA, T., FLOREEN, A. C. The dissatisfied patient with chronic pain. *Pain 4:* 367–377, 1978.
30. TOOMEY, T. C., GHIA, J. N., MAO, W., AND GREGG, J. M. Acupuncture and chronic pain mechanisms: The moderating effects of affect, personality and stress on response to treatment. *Pain 3:* 137–146, 1977.
31. TURK, D., AND GENEST, M. *Behavioural Group Therapy: Group Therapy for Pain.* Research Press, Yale University, New Haven, 1979.
32. WOLPE, J. *Psychotherapy by Reciprocal Inhibition.* Stanford University Press, Stanford, CA, 1958.
33. YALOM, I. D. *The Theory and Practice of Group Psychotherapy.* Basic Books, New York, 1975.
34. ZIMBARDO, P. G., COHEN, A. R., WEISENBERG, M., DWORKIN, L., AND FIRESTONE, I. Control of pain motivation by cognitive dissonance. In *Pain: Clinical and Experimental Perspectives,* edited by M. Weisenberg. St. Louis, 1975, pp. 166–170.

13

Psychiatric Management of Chronic Pain

ELDON TUNKS, M.D.

The Relevance of Psychiatry

In the past 30 years, and particularly in the past 10, there has been considerable development of models and techniques for the study and the management of chronic pain problems. Added to the already established body of psychiatric theory and technique, these newer ideas and applications provide a creative and relevant contribution that is welcome to the liaison-consultation psychiatrist.

Hypnotic methods, of course, are rather old as far as the modern psychiatric era is concerned, but there has been a revived interest in them in the matter of pain treatment. A number of apparently contrasting points of view are found. Some regard hypnotic phenomena as a function of various mental structures and levels of awareness, some as a function of cues and expectancies, and others in terms of information processing and communication patterns (1, 21, 47, 71). The proponents of all of these points of view, however, have elucidated valuable strategies that can be applied to chronic pain; rather than being contradictory, these various approaches appear to complement each other.

In the 1960s there was a great growth of interest in the behavior therapies as an alternative to other mental models. Fordyce and his co-workers (15) describe the application of operant conditioning methods to the treatment of chronic pain patients. Following the publication of impressive results documented by this group, similar programs were established in many other places, supporting the value of such an approach (5–7, 46, 48, 50, 60). Relevant as this approach is, it is not always an available alternative for a psychiatric consultant who would require the assistance of a psychologist and a multidisciplinary rehabilitation team to put such a program into effect. Such programs also raise some doubts because, at least in their description, they appear mechanical and lacking in emphathy and possibly, therefore, inimical to the therapeutic alliance that the psychiatrist wishes to establish with his client.

There has been much recent interest in the development of cognitive-behavioral approaches (2, 33, 66, 67; Cameron, Chapter 7 this volume). Although based on behavioral theory, these approaches lend themselves to both individual and group application and can be adapted to psychiatric practice.

Studies of the effect of modeling on behavior are not new (52), but the use of modeling strategies in pain has been examined in detail by Craig and his co-workers (8, 9). There is particular merit in understanding the principle of modeling for anyone dealing with clinical pain. It is obvious, for example, that chronic pain patients may be detrimentally influenced by other family members who also demonstrate illness behavior (43, 50). Much of the therapeutic efficacy of group treatments may well depend on modeling (Baptiste and Herman, Chapter 12 this volume). The therapeutic milieu can be deliberately organized to provide an environment for treatment of chronic pain patients (17, 68). In the practice of psychiatric consultation to a rehabilitation setting, individual patient problems are often directly related to ward atmosphere through the effects of direct observation and modeling, and sometimes intervention must be made at this level.

Helpful as these insights and applications are for interdisciplinary teams and pain clinics, the psychiatrist who consults to medical, surgical or rehabilitation wards and clinics is himself apt to be asked to see a large number of patients who suffer both pain and psychological disturbance. Questions posed may relate to whether there is a psychological etiology for the problem, whether a psychological management is appropriate and whether there exist psychosocial complications of the chronic disorder. At times the referral will be made not because of the patient's complaint but because family members or staff are disturbed by the patient's behavior. For many patients referred, their psychological distress is partly a result of their intractable pain (38). For many others, their complaint of pain arises because of psychological problems (10, 11, 25, 39, 55, 59).

What the psychiatrist in particular brings to bear in such cases relates in part to his training and in part to specific skills needed for this sort of work. His medical/neurological training and language enable him to appreciate the background of the problem from the point of view of the medical system and enable him to translate this understanding into terms the patient can comprehend. At the same time, there is familiarity with patterns of psychiatric distress and disorder, biological treatments for such problems, and at least one psychodynamic model for intervention at the individual, family, or group level. Particular information and skills that must be used to effectively deal with the chronic pain patient include familiarity with assessment and management of psychological problems in the disabled (4) and literature relevant to the psychiatric discipline in management of pain (19, 27, 35, 58, 64). It would be helpful if the psychiatrist used a terminology that avoids confusion (36), avoiding, as well, unhelpful distinctions such as "'psychogenic" versus "true organic pain."

There are three levels at which a psychiatrist may be expected to provide expertise. Direct assessment, consultation and treatment are the most common requests, as in the rest of medicine. Patients themselves, likewise, usually expect direct contact and assistance from the consultants as with other medical specialists. Some consultative work is directed toward team functioning. It is usually case-oriented because of the problems particular patients present, the need to understand the psychological dynamics of patient behavior, and the need to develop methods of treatment. Nonpsychiatric staff may also require skills such as interviewing, recognizing psychiatric signs and symptoms, and handling psychotropic drugs. Thus, frequently the psychiatrist has a role in education and administration with respect to pain management—this usually occurring in the context of a chronic pain clinic or rehabilitation facility. It might be recognized that the psychiatrist has very appropriate skills for dealing simultaneously with medical and psychological concepts, and it is not surprising that a number of psychiatrists have found it suitable to administer or give leadership in chronic pain and rehabilitation programs.

Consultation in a Nonpsychiatric Setting

On the medical or surgical ward, the implications of the very admission of a patient serves usually to reinforce a "body-mind dichotomy." The psychiatrist seems like an intruder, and psychological interventions may appear irrelevant to the patient with pain. A psychiatric consultant is usually brought in on the same basis as other medical consultants—being asked to interview, conduct specific examinations and provide a diagnosis. This means he is part of the medical milieu and likely subscribes to the medical disease model (49). Faced with the prospect of seeing a psychiatrist, the patient may be tempted to feel defensive, as if being accused that his pain is "psychological" rather than "real." A specific rehabilitation ward may mitigate against this sort of incompatibility because of a greater tendency on such units to use a multidisciplinary approach from the beginning and to concentrate on adjustment as well as on recovery. In many cases, however, the space for rheumatology, orthopaedics, and rehabilitation is shared so that a "rehabilitation atmosphere" may not fully develop. The patient may feel confused also by the multiple modalities of treatment he may be receiving; injection of steroids, physiotherapy, and prescription of a brace might all imply disease, whereas visits by the social worker and occupational therapist and consultation with the psychiatrist might imply to him that the staff no longer believe in his disability.

As suggested above, the clinical setting itself may have a great deal to do with how the patient perceives his problem. If many other patients are physically ill and receiving a heavy input of medical care, the pain patient may well expect he needs the same. Exposed to dissatisfied or anxious patients, the pain sufferer may similarly experience dissatisfaction and anxiety (8). In determining the nature of the problem, therefore, the psychiatrist usually must depend not only on the basic medical report and his own observations and interview but also on staff impressions and reports and observations of the ward itself.

As mentioned, the problem must be evaluated in its context. Patients will report to the psychiatrist what they believe is relevant; they may withhold information bearing on family or social dysfunction because, as they see it, this has nothing to do with their pain problem and may give a wrong impression. To validate his impressions of the patient, the psychiatrist is well-advised to ask for an interview with other family members or the spouse. A number of studies have shown an important link between the behavior of pain patients, illness or complaints in other family members, and the outcome of the treatment process (29, 43, 48, 50, 53). Occasionally there is considerable resistance by the patient to the suggestion that another family member ought to be included. There are two ways in which this resistance can be lessened. Where there is a policy to carry out a psychosocial assessment routinely for all new patients, spouses or family members can be included from the first so that the patient does not feel alarmed when the psychiatrist later makes a similar request to see the family. A simple explanation is also quite helpful, such as, "We find that problems such as yours, which have lasted a long time, have in some ways involved everyone in the family. Now that we are going to start making things better we will need everyone's help. I am sure you have all wanted to be of help to each other in this problem but didn't know where to begin."

A fourth problem faced by the consultant is that the patient is referred, but it may be someone other than the patient who is manifesting the discomfort. When another medical specialist such as a cardiologist is called in, one readily assumes that the patient himself experiences distress and is asking for a solution. In the matter of psychiatric referrals, however, it may occur that the patient does not identify himself as having a problem, but rather that a family member has complained to staff or that staff are running into difficulty with behavior that they view as disruptive or maladaptive. Examples of this would be the patient who remains in bed, not participating in treatments because of pain, or the family member who calls staff concerning the amount of medication the ill member appears to be taking at home. Not infrequently, staff on a nonpsychiatric unit may ask the psychiatrist to see someone in the hope that the patient will be transferred to another "more appropriate" (psychiatric) service; such referrals may indicate that a negative countertransference or other unpleasant feelings are being stirred up in the staff, who may feel powerless to deal with it. Although the patient may require attention, solving such problems often requires that time be spent with nursing and other staff, helping them express the frustrations they feel in a certain situation and helping them develop models, strategies, and skills so that they themselves can cope with the patient (51).

Psychiatric Management of Chronic Pain

ATTITUDE

All too often, patients may expect to be blamed or disbelieved by a psychiatrist. The experienced consultant will anticipate such feelings even before he encounters the patient and will demonstrate a manner that is empathic and an attitude that is "client-centered." After introducing himself and before proceeding further, the consultant should ascertain that the patient knew about and was prepared for the visit. Ensuring the patient's sense of privacy, providing a position in which the patient can be comfortable and being aware of his sitting tolerance and need to change position are important in conveying empathy, as is taking adequate time to review the progress and status of his medical condition. It is usually profitable to the psychiatrist, and reassuring to the patient, to complete the interview by an appropriate physical examination which may be confined to the body system or area of complaint. Toward the end of an interview, patients are usually gratified to have the consultant briefly summarize, without jargon, what has been learned and to be invited to voice any questions and to agree with the psychiatrist on what should be the next step in intervention (34; Pilowsky, Chapter 8 this volume).

PROBLEM ANALYSIS

At this point, most clinicians recognize the fallacy of the "body-mind dichotomy." What is not so easy is defining a conceptual framework in which a chronic pain problem can be more appropriately formulated (Chapter 2). The most acceptable solution to this problem in recent years has been the adoption of some sort of multidimensional or multiaxial framework (64). A simple framework for formulation, for example, might follow the lines of the DSM-III. Even more simply, pain might be considered as having biological, psychological, and social dimensions. As a biological event, pain is seen as a signal subserved by central and peripheral processing systems that are tied both to sensory and to cognitive and motivational systems (26). Simultaneously, pain is a psychological phenomenon with cognitive and affective import (3). The very fact that pain presents clinically to some other individual demonstrates that it is also a social event with communication value (61). The relative importance of these various axes or dimensions may differ from case to case, but all are relevant all the time. Of further importance is the use of a language and terminology which does not lead to ambiguity (36).

Having formulated the problem in this manner, the clinician must deal with several other questions. What is the reasonable outcome of intervention, or what is the likely outcome of rehabilitation? Expectations must take into account factors such as age, social support, intelligence and skill levels, duration of illness or unemployment, and irreversible medical changes. Following from this question comes the next, "Can a common focus for therapeutic endeavor be agreed upon?" Too many psychiatric consultations end with a statement that "the patient is, unfortunately, not psychologically minded" and is, therefore, unsuitable for therapy. A more helpful approach to the problem is to determine what the patient is in fact prepared to do. As an example, a patient will sometimes state that he can accept nothing less than pain relief and that he does not see his problem in psychological terms. In reply, the interviewer can ask the patient to consider the "hypothetical" case that his pain, when all is said and done, might be incompletely relieved. This can open up a line of discussion leading to a fruitful shared focus. Care must be taken at the same time to ensure that the focus chosen by the patient is realistic. Patients may overreach or underreach their grasp and this must be pointed out to them.

The third question to be posed is, "What environmental changes are necessary for the individual to change his behavior? Furthermore, what will be the impact on the patient's natural environment if change does occur?" It seems almost trite to say it, but patients not only come to the hospital because they are sick but also, in some ways, may be sick because they come to the hospital. To make people well, therapists may have to modify their own responses to their patient. Even this is probably insufficient if, at the same time, members of the patient's family and significant others are not also taught new ways of responding so that illness behavior will no longer be perpetuated (14, 29). Failures in rehabilitation can often be traced to a family environment which has promoted unhealthy attitudes or to a lack altogether of adequate family or social support so that incentives for well behavior are too meagre (48, 50).

ALIGNING STRATEGY TO PROBLEM ANALYSIS

Strategies have to be tailored to the problem at hand. Some strategies focus more on relationship to the individual and others more on the environment.

In *working with the individual patient* the first step is to identify the "case manager," who may be the attending physician or the therapist playing a pivotal role in the treatment process. Notwithstanding the psychiatric consultant's relationship with the patient, this case manager has to be perceived as centrally involved in the rendering of opinion and in the ratification of all treatment plans. In addition, misconceptions and frightful fantasies by the patient about what is really wrong have to be uncovered and rectified. This is best done by reviewing the positive findings in a simple way with him. There is a tendency, which must be avoided, to put some things in negative terms only (e.g., "After all our tests we have found there is nothing wrong with you to explain your pain"). The author has often found it useful to coach the attending physician on how to present information to the patient, modeling the interview but leaving it to the attending physician to carry it out. Again, for the sake of simplicity, the information to be given to the patient can be divided into biological, psychological, and social categories. An example of an explanation might be illustrated as follows:

Case Report

A 25-year-old man with a poor work history and a turbulent childhood complained of arthritis all over his body. Investigation in the Rheumatic Disease Unit found him to be operating at a markedly disabled level but with no evidence of articular or rheumatic disease. The report given to the patient ran something like this:

We admitted you because you had been suffering a great deal of pain and had been unable to work for nearly a year. While observing you in hospital, we certainly confirmed that your level of activity is very poor, to the point where your home life is suffering, in addition to the fact that you are unemployed. We think your inability to sleep is probably important in your problem. Fortunately, we see that you are not suffering from any progressive arthritis or crippling disease, and your muscles, joints and nervous system can be capable of quite healthy function given the proper chance. You do not need to let your pains alarm you into making you believe that you are as sick as you sometimes feel. The sleep disturbance you have is very likely part of the discouraged mood you have been describing; the fear you expressed initially that something awful was happening to your body, I am sure, did not help either. You have told us about the great discomfort you have suffered, and we remember also that you told us that your job was in jeopardy and your financial security is threatened, and you just have not been able to enjoy yourself with other people the way you remember you used to. We have seen many people with this sort of problem. Some people call it "fibrositis" or "nonarticular rheumatism," which really boils down to saying that you have pain in certain places in your body but without any damage being done. Some sorts of pain, as you know, get much better by resting, as when you sprain your ankle. Other kinds of pain do not, and you certainly have proven that to yourself because with all of your resting things have only gotten worse. The surprising thing about this sort of pain is that it gets better with physical activity and improved fitness if this is carried out in a regular supervised manner. We are going to help you with this program as well as teach you some methods for relaxing and getting to sleep at night. We do not plan to ignore your concerns, either, about what is happening at home and can meet with you and your family about that, regularly, until things get sorted out. You probably would like to know that it will be possible for you to return to your usual job in the near future without any risk or harm to yourself, although you may have some residual pain problems from time to time, for example, with weather changes. You will probably feel a good deal better with your fitness program and with the additional help of a relaxation training program and a prescription which you might take at night.

People need explanations when they are threatened in some way—giving the problem a name seems to be half the battle in reducing their anxiety. Jargon names, however, may convey something to professionals but will probably mystify patients, who are much happier to have their problem described to them in operational terms, as with the example above. Frank (16) has called this "satisfying the principle of Rumpelstiltskin."

Patients often see themselves as victims of their pain and see their pain as an infliction or invasion. Helping them to "accept ownership" of their problem can be a large conceptual leap. In the course of an interview the patient can be led to see how he has actively participated in the changes that have occurred in his life, entertaining fantasies, seeking inappropriate solutions, fighting losing battles and so forth. He will readily agree if he is told that no one has the right to judge the severity or validity of the pain but the patient himself, and from this he can be led to see that his coping has always been his business too. An agreement for intervention can then be set out, which may take the form of an explicit contract or may be expressed informally in terms of mutual expectations. Having identified the focus that the patient is willing to share with the therapist and having discussed expectations for therapeutic outcome, the clinician can outline a course of action directly engaging the patient on his own behalf as a full participant in the therapy. To be successful, the therapeutic strategy must show a good fit between the therapist's and the patient's understanding of the problem. The focus of intervention, expectations for outcome, and the therapy itself should be marked by a high level of involvement of and support from the therapist, a high degree of apparent relevance to the pain problem, and palatability, including opportunities for face-saving if that is necessary (37). In this therapeutic process the psychiatrist may take the role of a primary therapist or may choose to give active support to the other case manager or attending physician.

The other component of strategic intervention involves *clinical teamwork and environmental intervention.* If one accepts that the environment can foster and perpetuate illness behavior by the nature of environmental responses, then it follows as well that illness behavior might be changed by altering environmental responses. A good place to begin this is with clinical staff. This may take the form of assisting nonpsychiatric staff to become more therapeutic in a psychological sense (51) or may go so far as to create a treatment team specialized in the behavioral management of pain (14, 57, 58). In any event, whatever the explicit programming, it is of tremendous advantage if the psychiatrist can make clinical rounds, so that his presence in the ward or clinic is seen to be natural. This heightens the level of awareness that the staff will have for behavioral and psychological issues and provides a ready and practical forum for education. The time invested initially is more than repaid by the improved working relationship and the increased therapeutic sophistication that the staff will show.

Nurses and other nonpsychiatric staff often have difficulties at first in grasping the diverse concepts distinguishing the treatment of acute pain from the management of chronic pain. Although it must be agreed that divisions such as "operant" versus "respondent" and "chronic" versus "acute" may be difficult to make at times, there is a certain heuristic value in using these categories in an educational program (57). One of the most common reasons for reluctance in dealing with psychological problems in a nonpsychiatric setting is the feeling that the staff sometimes have of being unskilled—of feeling at a loss when confronted with a difficult patient. Having some conceptual model by which to describe the problem they are dealing with and some basic ideas of the sort of intervention that would be appropriate makes a great deal of difference in how successfully staff in a nonpsychiatric setting can deal with psychological disturbance. It needs to be emphasized that nurses in particular occupy a pivotal role in the delivery of health care. They spend the largest amount of time with the patients and are the ones who have the greatest opportunities for longitudinal observation, and it is to them that the patient will usually go first when in distress. The nursing staff, then, are at the heart of the therapeutic atmosphere of a unit.

With regard to therapeutic atmosphere, it is not a new idea to psychiatry to manage an inpatient unit along the lines of group functioning and to deliberately construct a "therapeutic milieu" in which the patients take an active participating role. It is valuable to recognize that the therapeutic milieu in a formal sense probably operates indirectly in most successful "behavior modification units" that deal with chronic pain. Furthermore, there have been a few reports of the establishment of successful inpatient treatment programs for chronic pain that were modeled along the line of the therapeutic milieu as an alternative to the more classical format of the operant conditioning model (17, 68). Whereas the operant conditioning model may appear authoritarian and lacking in empathy, the therapeutic milieu, by giving greater emphasis to group functioning and group responsibility for program outcome, may be a more palatable format while still allowing for an element of contingency management using mostly social reinforcers and the effects of modeling.

A technique used by many involved with chronic pain treatment is the therapeutic "contract" (15, 18). In a typical "contract" a reasonable set of therapeutic outcomes is spelled out in detail. There also is a clear delineation of what sort of action is required both from the client and also from the staff if that therapeutic outcome is to be achieved. An example of a contract for pain treatment is shown in Figure 13.1. The contract is usually comple-

<u>CONTRACT FOR TREATMENT</u>

<u>PAIN PROGRAM</u>

NAME: _____

DATE OF
ADMISSION: _____

I request admission to the Pain Program of Chedoke Hospital for a period of
_____weeks. The objectives of my admission are:

☐ prevocational assessment

☐ to increase my ability to be active while at home ____hours per day

☐ to return to my previous job

☐ to go to a lighter job ____hours per day _____

☐ to help me (or my family) to get along better

☐ to control my medication and reduce harmful amounts of medications

☐ to have the following treatments to help reduce my discomfort

             - relaxation training
             - exercise in pool

               _____

               _____

               _____

☐

☐

I will remain in the treatment program for the agreed duration of
treatment, unless mutually agreed by myself and treatment staff.

I will participate in all scheduled activities even though my pain may
continue to present some problem.

Treatment staff agree to make available to me all elements of the
Rehabilitation Program as explained to me and to discuss with me, my
progress at regular intervals, including making suggestions that may
assist me in achieving my goals.

Patient Signature: _____ Date: _____

Therapist Signature: _____

mented by a system of charting and self-monitoring. If a contract is properly drawn up, it can provide a useful tool in negotiating difficulties that occur.

Case Report

A patient being treated for chronic low back pain failed to get up from his bed to go to scheduled activities. A member of the nursing staff visited the patient in his room and heard the patient's complaint that the pain was too severe and that, for this reason, the patient was unable to get out of bed. The nurse recalled the contract that the patient had drawn up with the staff and reasoned this way:

"You can't get up because your pain is too severe?"

"Yes."

"What was it like before you got into hospital?"

"Oh, the same sort of thing. Sometimes I'd have a better day and could do some things, but on days like today I'd stay in bed—maybe 2–3 days at a time if the pain really got bad like it is now."

"You were really stuck."

"Mmmm."

"What do you hope to accomplish by being in this rehabilitation unit?"

"I was hoping they would make me better, but the things they are having me do just make me hurt more."

"But isn't that the problem you were having at home? On the good days you would do what you could and on the bad days you couldn't do anything. If you use the same strategy here in hospital, of doing what you feel like on the good days and nothing at all on the bad days, how is that really any different from at home? What do you think you could learn that would be any different?"

"Well, what should I do about the pain?"

"In your contract with us you agreed that since your pain has been chronic and wasn't better with rest that you would attempt to improve your physical stamina and fitness, pain or no pain. We promised that doing that would not be harmful to you and that if you really followed through on it, at the very least, you would achieve more independence, and very likely you would be a lot happier with yourself and probably more comfortable too. If we are going to deliver what we promised, then it seems you will have to deliver what you promised."

Design of a Therapeutic Milieu

At times, it is possible to set up a treatment module for management of people with chronic pain. This does not have to be a whole ward by itself but should at least involve a large enough number of beds to create a working group of patients and should allow the patients to be situated in such a way that they will have close working contact and be able to influence each other. A therapeutic milieu must operate around a basic philosophy which must be promoted by group education. A consistent group of staff members is essential—those familiar with this sort of method of managing chronic pain. Previous exposure to a psychiatric unit may be helpful to the staff. The therapeutic milieu for chronic pain patients, however, is not simply a psychiatric program and must involve a number of activities relevant to the person with chronic pain. Education regarding back care, the use of medication, body mechanics, stress and other relevant topics must be interspersed with group sessions in which patients are invited to express their feelings. Occupational therapy, placement in workshops, a fitness program supervised by a physiotherapist, and relaxation programs all are valuable and usually should be carried out with the group format. Contact must be maintained with the families, and occasionally more intensive family therapy is necessary. Sometime early in the hospitalization, contact must be made with agencies and employers who will be continuing with the patient after he is discharged, to ensure a smooth transition away from the hospital. Overall, patients can be meaningfully engaged in working toward a set of reasonable goals, once these have been negotiated with the staff, can profitably take responsibility for monitoring and achieving the outcome, and can share the responsibility with each other in the patients' group. This approach is mentioned here in brief form with the further comment that patients who participate in such a program generally find this sort of program high in apparent relevance, palatability and empathy.

Other Treatment Methods

GROUP TREATMENTS

Baptiste and Herman (Chapter 12 this volume) discuss the use of groups in some detail. There are many types of group therapy that have been found useful in management of chronic pain (7, 17, 20, 46). It should be noted, however, that pain patients cannot easily be introduced into a group of psychiatric patients and, similarly, psychiatric patients may be rejected by a group of chronic pain patients. As mentioned above, the group format may be an essential element in the functioning of an inpatient pain program. Transactional analysis is favored by some to deal with "pain games" (17). Another possible variation brings together patients and their spouses. Even "alumni" groups have been formed of patients who have been discharged from a pain program (46). Group education programs are becoming a common service in physiotherapy departments and in pain clinics. Typically, these use a classroom and practical demonstration approach to body mechanics and posture, usually with emphasis on the low back, and may include instruction in general relaxation. Although, on the face of it, these educational groups explicitly address the need for information, it is clear that modeling and other group dynamics also operate to make them therapeutic. The psychiatrist might have a role in supervising such groups or in being one of several professional contributors.

RELAXATION TRAINING

Relaxation techniques may not be seen as falling within the usual job description of the psychiatrist, but they are so useful and widely used for chronic pain that the consultant may well employ them himself or supervise someone else in their application. Relaxation training itself can be quite effective in pain control (24, 42) and there is good reason to believe that, in most cases, hypnosis and biofeedback, which are much more complex and difficult procedures to carry out, provide, by and large, no better results. Whether disorders like low back and neck pain are actually due to chronic muscle "spasms" probably is in some doubt even though this "spasm" is at times associated with the chronic pain, either as a cause or as an effect. Learning to relax, however, improves the sense of mastery, reduces the sense that stress is overwhelming, and may provide an occasion for learning cognitive strategies for pain control.

THE PSYCHOTHERAPIES

Psychotherapy in its various forms is discussed elsewhere in this book (Chapters 7–12). Most psychiatrists are familiar with at least one system of psychotherapy. If the explicit motive of the psychotherapy is complete relief of pain, however, the results are often unsatisfactory. More reasonable goals include the alleviation of emotional distress, improvement in interpersonal function and self-esteem, and improved adjustment to disability. One encounters occasional cases in which psychotherapy alone has been employed with great success for someone with chronic pain, but such cases are in the minority.

PSYCHOTROPIC MEDICATION

There are two aspects to psychotropic management for chronic pain patients. The first is that harmful side effects should be eliminated. Narcotics, sedatives, hypnotics and many of the drugs that chronic pain patients use in combination have the effect of reducing motivation and of creating apathy, depression and irritability or other unpleasant states of mind. Nevertheless, patients are unwilling to give up these medications unless they are given an opportunity to become educated as to what drugs do and to learn about the rational use of medication. In some cases it is necessary to provide a treatment setting in which patients can withdraw from drugs to which they have become dependent (7, 15, 46). One regime for medication reduction is the sort described by Fordyce (14). On an inpatient basis, narcotics and habituating sedatives are given in a liquid constant volume and masked with a flavor to make it difficult to taste the contents. Medication is then given regularly, usually every 4 hours rather than on an as needed basis for pain. This timing conforms to the average biological life of most analgesics so that a steady blood level is maintained and the pain cycle is not reestablished before each new dose. Over a period of time, the contraindicated medications are withdrawn and replaced perhaps with antipyretic analgesics or maybe with psychotropic drugs. Sedatives and narcotics can almost always be withdrawn without making the patient worse, and usually making the patient better.

While some medications may be harmful in chronic pain, others may be of benefit. Antidepressants such as amitriptyline and the tricyclic group of drugs may exert at least some of their effect by relieving concurrent depression (65). There may also be a direct effect on the nociceptive neurological systems in some cases, so that antidepressants used properly may bring about useful pain relief after a period of a few days (40, 62). The postulated mechanism of action of the antidepressant group of drugs is prevention of reuptake of neurotransmitter from the synaptic cleft, in this way increasing the concentration of neurotransmitter at the synapse and increasing the probability of neurotransmission. Serotonin may have a specific role in pain perception, linked to the endorphin system. Tricyclic antidepressants have shown their value in conditions such as migraine, fibrositis syndrome, and atypical facial neuralgia as well as in giving non-specific benefit to chronic pain patients with sleep disorders and problems associated with increased muscle tension.

Phenothiazines are occasionally valuable, although usually in association with antidepressants, in such problems as neuralgia, causalgia, and thalamic syndrome.

The greatest difficulty in the use of psychotropic drugs is that they are often given in inappropriate doses. Beginning at too high a dosage level may cause alarming side effects which will make the patient thereafter reject the drug. It is usually helpful to begin with a low dose before bedtime, gradually increasing it as the patient tolerates it at a rate sufficient that sleep is improved but that morning wakening is unimpaired. Adequate doses are also necessary, and it is increasingly possible for therapeutic blood levels to be ascertained. For most adults the dosage range of amitriptyline that may be effective is between 50 and 150 mg taken mostly at night. For phenothiazines the dosages differ depending on the substance, but an example would be from 2 mg to 8 mg perphenazine taken mostly at night.

Although they do not come under the class of psychotropic drugs, it is often forgotten that antipyretic analgesics can be very effective if used properly in regular but not excessive dosages. Although pain relief from antipyretics is modest, it is reliable and, in most cases, without serious side effect.

Integrating Medical and Psychiatric Approaches

It has been advocated elsewhere (18) that holistic approaches are desirable and possible, integrating both the medical and the psychological dimensions; an example might illustrate this.

Transcutaneous electrical nerve stimulation was carried out as a regular service in a local physiotherapy department. Therapeutic results had been rather good for a period of time with one certain experienced therapist, but it was noted that some other newer therapists were using the same devices in apparently the same way but were getting much less effective results. An on-site visit led to the observation that the first therapist had the habit of beginning with a new patient by asking the patient if he knew what this treatment was all about. She then would give a brief statement of the rationale for electrical stimulation, linking the patient's pain with an explanation of counterirritation and the effects on the nervous system. The patient was reassured that no harm would come from use of the device and that taking time to relax before the treatments often improved the results. The patient was also told that his active cooperation was required since accurate reporting and adjustment of the device was what made the treatment effective. Other therapists had been taking much more of a "scientific" attitude, not wanting to "prejudice" the patient. They were offering the device as something which may or may not be beneficial but were noting that the actual mechanisms of TNS had never been proven and that, since the device was costly, it would be important that the patient answer exactly whether he was improved by it or whether he merely thought he was improved. Time was spent showing physiotherapy staff how positive expectations were a reasonable and important part of any treatment, and some role-playing was done to work out a routine that the staff would be comfortable with in speaking with patients. Following this, it was noticed that the results of electrical stimulation improved considerably.

Under discussion here is the "nonspecific psychotherapeutic effects" that may be found in any number of treatments. These involve elements such as expectation, enhanced motivation, increased activity, and other factors which might be described loosely as "placebo effect," but which are, in fact, an essential part of any effective therapy that actively involves the patient (16). Being aware of these factors and actively manipulating them can greatly improve outcome.

Case Examples

Problems of chronic pain are diverse and examples are offered not to provide a comprehensive tally of every possible permutation but rather to provide illustration of the material discussed so far.

MEDICATION ABUSE

It is not always easy to define when the use of a certain drug is good or bad. Generally, in chronic pain, however, sedatives, hypnotics and opiates are not particularly useful long-term, and the longer the usage continues the more likely it is that tolerance will develop. This in itself is not directly a problem, but escalation of dosage may lead to multiplication of other unwanted effects, such as impairment of thinking, mood, and motivation, and all of this may provoke anxiety not only in the physician, who may be reluctant to prescribe these medications, but also in concerned others, including the family. When a patient is admitted and has been accustomed to receiving high doses of such medications, the physicians and other staff may express concern about addiction or medication abuse. Even more so, concern is aroused when it is seen that patients have incorporated the use of a medication into a pattern of chronic illness behavior—in this case, the overuse of a particular drug serving as a defense against anxiety or other unpleasant feelings. The discontinuation of drugs that are proving to be problematic is a major goal of pain treatment. It should be remembered that, at times, the reduction and discontinuation of certain analgesics may actually improve pain control if the intake of the drug has been constant— this is often seen in the case of headaches and neuralgias that have been treated with excessive quantities of pills containing combinations of anti-pyretics and opiate.

Case Report

Mrs. A.B. This 55-year-old married woman had a 30-year history of chronic low back pain which had begun while she was riding on horseback but had progressed insidiously afterward. In the 10 years prior to being seen in our clinic she had had discectomies at L4-5 and L5-S1, a fusion from L5 to S1 and a laminectomy of L5-S1, with continued worsening in her pain complaint. She had been obtaining, from her family physician, prescriptions for meperidine and had eventually reached an intake of approximately 5.5 g/week, most of which she would use in the first 5 days and for the rest of the week would buy tablets containing ASA and 8 mg codeine and would take methyprylon in variable amounts. Her physician had cautioned her several times that her medication intake was excessive and had threatened to reduce it, but she would respond with tears or with veiled hints about suicide and the prescriptions would continue. Her posture was to complain that she really did not want to be taking all of these medications, but when any alternative was proposed she would retreat to demanding effective pain relief.

Her husband was a business man who had achieved only marginal success. For several years he had spent many hours at his business, attempting to keep it afloat. He would always readily show up for a conjoint interview with his wife but would show very little affect and would barely look at his wife during the interview. Yet, both of them denied they had any problem other than her chronic pain and he presented himself as an extraordinarily long-suffering and patient individual. Partly on the insistence of the family physician, Mrs. A.B. agreed to be admitted to an inpatient pain treatment unit that used operant conditioning principles, but she soon after discharged herself against medical advice and returned to her family doctor and to an even worse pattern of medication intake. After about a year she obtained a consultation from a neurosurgeon and enquired whether deep brain stimulation might provide a cure for her pain. This surgeon found insufficient objective findings on physical examination to support the degree of pain complaint. He was concerned about the abuse of medication and refused to consider the deep brain stimulation procedure. He instead recommended the patient be admitted again to the pain treatment unit. The patient refused this but along with her husband came up with a compromise proposal. She would have her meperidine replaced with methadone which would be allotted in decreasing amounts every week until she finally withdrew totally. The family arranged for her to spend her time at the family cottage while this was going on.

It became apparent that as the methadone allottments decreased, family members ran an increasing number of errands into town for Mrs. A.B. to pick up other extra medication, so that soon she was consuming approximately 50 methyprylon capsules and 200 tablets of ASA with codeine per week—8 mg codeine per tablet. She was found unconscious by the family and taken to the suicidology unit of the hospital, whence she was referred again to the pain treatment unit. She agreed this time to remain for 3 weeks. During her inpatient stay, her methadone was given to her in a masked solution of constant volume with a decreasing amount of methadone each day so that after 3 weeks the opiate was totally withdrawn. The patient steadfastly refused to participate in patient groups or discussions; at the time the medication had been completely withdrawn, she immediately discharged herself from hospital despite suggestions that she might receive further benefit from staying. She refused to return for follow-up or to answer inquiries.

"PSYCHOPHYSIOLOGICAL" PAIN SYNDROMES

Pain is often associated with unpleasant affective states, such as anxiety (41), depression (65) and resentment (38). The degree of unpleasant affect often correlates with pain. This is not to say that the pain is simply a manifestation of psychological conversion but that certain unpleasant affects may reasonably accompany pain as well as have a psychological and psychophysiological role in exacerbating the pain problem. Apart from the fact that low back pain, neuralgias, or any chronic pain problem has important implications for both physical and psychological functioning, a number of disorders seem to depend on an interaction or association between psychological and physiological derangement. Temporomandibular joint dysfunction or the myofacial pain-dysfunction syndrome (31) is almost always associated with states of tension or depression and habits of daytime or nighttime bruxism. Atypical facial neuralgia (12, 23, 28; Violon, Chapter 3 this volume) has long been recognized as a disorder in which psychiatric factors—particularly depression—are important. Fibrositis (44, 45), otherwise called the central panalgesia syndrome (54), involves a picture of chronic pain felt in particular muscle groups near the spine especially and in legs and arms, associated with nonrestorative sleep patterns and often depression or unpleasant mood. Psychiatrists may take a special interest in such syndromes because of the psychological signs associated.

Case Report

Mrs. C.D. This 25-year-old woman was accompanied by her husband to the Clinic, complaining of pain in her left ear. The pain had begun after the birth of the first child 1 year previously, about the same time that a friend was discovered to be suffering from a brain tumor and subsequently died. C.D. developed hyperventilation episodes, fears of going to sleep and fears of suffering from a brain tumor, and made a number of visits to emergency departments. Her father, who happened to be a physician, pointed out to her the psychological nature of her reaction and showed her how to relax and breathe into a paper bag; the hyperventilation syndrome disappeared, but the pain continued and she saw a series of dental and medical consultants. The pain itself was described as aching, stabbing and burning, as associated with a popping in her ears, and as worse with stress. When the pain was severe it was associated with phonophobia. She was anxious and irritable. Her husband noted that she was grinding her teeth while she slept. There was a family history of bruxism and migraines. She and her husband denied any family difficulties and stated that, despite her pain and medical visits, there was little in the way of disability. On physical examination she was tender in the posterior muscles of neck and shoulders, and there was evidence of temporomandibular joint dysfunction. There was hyperalgesia to pinprick on the left side of the scalp and face. The diagnosis was made of temporomandibular joint dysfunction associated possibly with atypical facial neuralgia. She was effectively managed with a prescription for amitriptyline, 75 mg taken at night, and a course of relaxation training taught to her by a physiotherapist.

Case Report

Mrs. E.F. This 40-year-old widow had an 8-year history of chronic pain, fatigue and insomnia. It was interesting to note that the patient's mother had also suffered pains and insomnia. E.F. was German-born, immigrating to Uruguay with her family as a young girl. She was the eldest of seven; her father was a laborer and her mother was frequently hospitalized with painful ailments. E.F. left school to obtain a job and help with the family income. She would commute home at night to look after her younger brothers and sisters. She found it difficult to get close to the father who was always working hard trying to make ends meet, and mother was inaccessible, either because she was hospitalized in a different town or because she was preoccupied with her own problems when she would return. She felt, however, that she had no right to ask any more from her parents who were suffering enough. She remembered as a young woman having had poor self-esteem and negative feelings about her own developing sexuality. As a teenager she experienced abdominal pains for several years. Married in her early twenties, she immigrated to Canada. Her husband was aggressive sexually and she was frightened of him. She believed that the demands of her religion would have her suffer his abuse, but she remembered lying awake many nights anticipating his late homecoming because there would be an argument, after which she might be beaten.

Eventually she developed a pattern of nonrestorative sleep, with difficulty getting to sleep and pains on awakening in the morning. The children became a discipline problem, with E.F. being mainly left with their care and her husband undermining her wishes. Her husband developed cancer and died, and E.F. found new friends and help from a social worker. As she became more assertive, she found that her children behaved themselves. When seen in the clinic, she was able to ventilate the resentment she had felt for many years, both against her parents and against her husband and members of her religion. She recognized that she had always attempted to hide her resentment or the expression of her need for understanding, even from herself, and that this was a lifelong pattern. Since she was already involved with helpful conversations in her hometown, the additional measures prescribed included amitriptyline to be taken at night, a fitness program to be supervised by a physiotherapy department, and referral to a government vocational and rehabilitation agency for retraining.

PAIN ASSOCIATED WITH MAJOR AFFECTIVE DISORDER

It has been observed that psychiatric patients quite frequently complain of pain (38). Pain complaints are relatively less frequent in the psychotic groups than among neurotics, but, nevertheless, psychoses may often include pain as an important presenting symptom. In many cases, no contributory causes are found and these pain experiences may represent hallucinations or distortions of physiologically based sensations, and they may be accompanied by delusional interpretations. At times, one encounters terms such as "depressive equivalent" or "masked depression." Such terms are unnecessarily ambiguous. It would seem preferable to identify the major psychiatric disorder which is, in fact, present on the basis of criteria which can be ascertained from history and mental status examination and inquiry into the family background.

Case Report

Mrs. G.H. This 26-year-old married woman came by herself to the clinic with a history of 3 years of pain which was gradually increasing in severity and spreading through her body. The pain would change in quality and migrate but particularly involved discomfort over one foot where she stated there was swelling and redness. She also complained of other symptoms such as numbness, tingling and dropping things from her hands; this symptom too was migrating. She was a nurse but had left her work some time before and, at the time of being seen, was pregnant for the second time. At interview she was fearful that some calamitous disease was being missed, was irritable, sad and anxious, and had symptoms of insomnia, fatigue, diurnal variation in her mood, poor appetite and tendency to social withdrawal. She felt that her thoughts were racing and her concentration was poor. There was no loosening of associations, delusion or hallucination in the formal sense. Physical examination carried out at the time found no abnormality, including the area where she said her foot was swollen and red. It was concluded that she was suffering from an affective disorder, although other possible causes for her pain were not considered to have been ruled out and she was treated with an antidepressant. On follow-up, it was noted that there was significant improvement. After that, there were occasional follow-up visits. She returned again, but without pain, about 3 years after the first assessment. She reported that she had had a third pregnancy, that her husband had left her immediately afterward, and that his leaving was a total surprise to her. This time her presentation was completely without pain symptoms but with symptoms of anxiety and panic, fears of catastrophe, and the impression that she was being followed, that she was hearing her thoughts broadcast on television, that she could hear her own thoughts spoken out loud and the feeling as if her thoughts were being withdrawn from her head. Being a nurse, she was able to say that she knew her disorder must be "paranoid" and that she needed help. She had difficulty keeping her thoughts on track and it was found that she had a flight of ideas but no loosening of associations. Treatment prescribed included moderate doses of amitriptyline and trifluoperazine to which she responded with resolution of her mood and thought disorder, and she thereafter benefited from ongoing counseling with a social worker.

THE "NONPSYCHOLOGICALLY MINDED" PATIENT

The language of dynamic psychiatry is derived from studies in psychoanalysis with populations of individuals who regarded themselves as psychologically distressed—persons with neuroses or personality disorders.

This language, although useful for some patient groups, is not necessarily always appropriate for patients who perceive themselves as suffering from bodily ailments. This is not to say that pain patients are not willing to gain insight, but rather that they are apt to respond more to an approach that is "client-centered" and is more apparently relevant to their distress. Patients who perceive themselves as ill need some demonstration of activity on the part of the therapist and must themselves also be actively engaged in the treatment process. The traditional psychotherapy model, therefore, may move too slowly for them. A further issue is that persons who have developed pain may tend to idealize their premorbid state and deny any problem other than the pain itself as being responsible for the predicament (69).

Case Report

This 49-year-old married woman was seen as an inpatient on a rheumatic disease unit because of her problem of rheumatoid arthritis. The staff had been concerned that her complaints were out of proportion to any demonstrable pathology. Mrs. I.J. showed excessive concern about physical symptoms and medications. Her children, now grown, reported to the staff that their mother had become very dependent and centered her whole existence on pain. She was seen with her husband and the couple denied any difficulties between them, although they admitted that he had had trouble with alcohol at some point. Mrs. I.J. did not see the point of psychiatric interventions. Help was offered but was not accepted and, shortly after, the patient was discharged.

A year later she was readmitted and was referred again because of the same concerns from the staff. The patient now revealed that in the intervening time she had separated from her husband because of his continued alcohol abuse, but that he still continued to visit her and that she was still cooking and washing for him. Again, she denied being in any distress except for the pain which prevented her from carrying out her physiotherapy and other assignments. A meeting, therefore, was held with ward staff, and the following strategy was drafted. The attending physician was to take time with the patient to explain that some pains are better with rest, but that some chronic pains do not respond and, instead, get worse if the person rests. For such pain, it is necessary to become active in the things that have been abandoned. She was asked to draw up a list of goals that she would like to achieve "if she were perfectly well," and when a list had been drawn up it was put in chart form and she was made responsible for charting her progress toward achieving these functional goals. For the first time, there was an improvement in her mood and in her level of activity and she was proud to show the progress she was now making. She spontaneously asked for a repeat visit to the psychiatrist. She had been doing a lot of thinking, she said, and was now aware of certain patterns he had ignored before. Her whole family had always done for others rather than being able to identify their own needs. Her upbringing had been austere and she had never felt comfortable in expressing her needs on her own behalf. She married a husband who was a "mamma's boy." The mother-in-law continually made excuses for him and expected I.J. to do the same. The in-laws blamed her when the husband drank excessively. She recognized that the only legitimate complaint she could ever make was that of being ill. The pattern was that she would push herself to the point where she felt she could not go any further; then she would develop symptoms and, only then, would feel that she had the attention rightfully owing to her. She agreed to an interview with her two children, who expressed their anxiety to their mother that she might continue in her old ways. They were concerned that she had the ability to control the whole family through her symptoms. She recognized their concerns and discussed alternate means of understanding communications and they agreed on cues to break these patterns of illness communication. All family members were relieved, and when she was discharged she no longer identified pain as a serious problem.

THE PROBLEM OF THE PATIENT WHO "COPES WELL"

Steger and Brockway (57) discuss the problem of the "stoic" individuals who, to the casual observer, appear to be doing well and to be heroic, but who have not been able to make appropriate adjustments since developing a disability. To those around them, they may present an image of strength or even be seen as admirable. There is no doubt that at times this sort of adjustment has merit, but the disadvantage is that more appropriate behavioral repertoires in line with their problems have not been developed. They also feel an obligation to be immune to the problem. Such persons may come from a family system where a sense of altruism is high. They may feel a personal obligation not to impose their difficulties on the family, and the family members may feel likewise. The need for these people is to learn more appropriate adaptive responses, to learn to ventilate feelings rather than push themselves to the point of breakdown, and to set limits on themselves and others.

Case Report

Mrs. K.L. This 50-year-old married woman was seen alone on the Rheumatic Disease Unit at her own request. She was suffering from psoriatic arthritis. Her husband was a prominent figure and the family was well-known for philanthropic contributions. She had always been cooperative as a patient, never showing dissatisfaction. As she interpreted it, she was becoming uneasy because the children were growing up and leaving home. Friends of similar age, whose children were also leaving home, were making new life-styles for themselves, going on vacations and extended cruises, and getting into other activities, whereas she was being held back by her arthritis. She related that her sense of uneasiness had begun about a year before when she had been asked to speak to a large group on the topic of "living with arthritis." Her speech had met with much approval and publicity, but she noted that she began to resent the image she had of herself and that others had of her, of "coping so well."

She denied that there had ever been any serious family trouble. They had always been quiet, and disputes had been settled by a quiet process of reasoning. Should she express some dissatisfaction or distress, her husband would reassure her and would be apt to bring her a gift the next day. She surmised that she might deal with unpleasant feelings in a similar way. After discussion she began to realize that what she really wanted from her family was the knowledge that she could share not only positive but also vulnerable feelings and that this was particularly important for her in her relationship with her husband now that their children were growing up and leaving home. She recognized the tendency that both she and her husband had to protect each other's feelings and thought it best that she would, on her own, open up the discussion of these issues with her husband. Medication was not prescribed.

COMPENSATION

Compensation has long been considered an important factor in prolonging illness, by decreasing the incentive to do well and by providing tangible "secondary gain." Frequently the term "compensation neurosis" is applied to individuals who demonstrate chronicity and who are awaiting the results of litigation or who are receiving some compensation benefit that is contingent on their remaining ill. It is probably correct to believe that financial compensation systems help perpetuate chronic pain problems (13). Hohl (22), in a study of whiplash patients, found that the length of time that had elapsed since injury, the vigor with which treatment was applied, and the presence of litigation all were significant factors in prolonging symptoms after injury. Block et al. (5) reported that patients referred from medical sources had a better outcome in a behaviorally oriented program for chronic pain than did patients referred from agencies which provided compensation. On the other hand, Maruta et al. (32) determined a number of factors that appeared to adversely affect outcome and, among these, found that the existence of a compensation system did not significantly reduce the likelihood of good results. Titchener and Ross (63), in a chapter in the American Handbook of Psychiatry, observed that the notion of "compensation neurosis" was in some ways shallow, based sometimes on a faulty notion of the concept of secondary gain. It was observed that seeking compensation might just as easily be seen as an adaptive response to a dilemma, if one accepts the fact that psychological and personal impairments are as valid and important as physiological ones. On the balance of it, it is likely that there are patients for whom the existence of future financial gain is an important variable in the perpetuation of the complaint. These individuals, though, are not likely to be attempting to be deceitful but, in the majority of cases, see themselves as having been wronged and are seeking retribution. At times, the vigor with which they approach litigation involves anger displaced from previous relationships with significant others and, therefore, may seem unrealistic and out of proportion. Furthermore, there is another way in which compensation may adversely affect the prognosis. Patients in receipt of benefits usually receive little more than would allow a state of dependency at the subsistence level: this income is usually unstable and subject to bureaucratic errors and decisions made by unknown persons. This combined with the length of time that individuals often must wait for final settlements aggravates a sense of anxiety, anger and uncertainty. Contrary to the habit of some to delay treatment until compensation is settled, the author would strongly advise that whenever patients are willing to undergo appropriate intervention, the latter should not be delayed.

Case Report

Mr. M.N. This 52-year-old man was admitted to the Inpatient Pain Treatment Unit for the second time. He had been seen as an outpatient 6 years before with depression, marked illness complaints, dizziness, odd patterns of numbness, "pain all over," blurred vision and inability to work since an automobile accident about 10 years previously. He reported that at the time of the automobile accident, everything had been going for him. He had had a regular job in maintenance for a school board and, in addition to that, in the evenings had a janitorial service and had recently invested in a restaurant. He recalled that his energy had been tireless and that he was about to really make good when the accident occurred. He had been involved in a collision in which the fault was attributed to the other driver and afterwards was unable to carry on his restaurant business or manage the evening work of his janitorial service. Finally he was not even able to carry on his regular employment with the school board and was fired. His wife had gone to work and he had been in receipt of workmen's compensation benefits. He recalled that shortly before the accident in question there had in fact been another auto accident in which his car had left the road, but he believed that no injury had been done to him at that time.

From another source, who had known him prior to his accident, it was gathered that he may have been running into business trouble even before his two accidents, but Mr. N. steadfastly held that he would have been able to make it work if he had had the health to carry on. "When I was well, I could work 18 hours a day and feel good." At first, the patient was willing to entertain individual conversations with the psychiatrist but did not participate in other pain clinic programs. His litigation came to court and he was awarded a modest settlement which he felt was unjust, but which he accepted, and he made agreements to continue conversations with the psychiatrist. Driving home from the lawyer's office, the very day that he picked up the settlement from the litigation, he sustained another rear-end collision and he arrived in the clinic in a very agitated state, stating that his situation now certainly must be hopeless. Litigation was again commenced. Nevertheless, the patient was involved in inpatient pain treatment for a 6-week period with the object that of increasing his level of functioning to the point where, on discharge, he may be able to make use of a retraining program sponsored by the government. He went from virtually no activity at all to approximately 2-hr work tolerance, and during his inpatient treatment it was noted that he was continually revising his goals downward. Nevertheless, he felt he had improved enough that he could enjoy his personal life. Conjoint marital psychotherapy was attempted after discharge, but his wife came only once and frankly did not believe that all of this input was really worth it, given the fact that her husband was not making big changes. Attempts at rehabilitation in a therapeutic workshop failed with him as an outpatient, and 1 year later he had his second admission to the inpatient program. He recognized that the way things were going he had "nothing to lose," and his goal this time was much more specifically stated. It was that he would apply for one of two available part-time jobs that would require 5 hr of physical activity per day after discharge. He entered the inpatient program, this time participated much more vigorously and achieved a 6-hr physical tolerance level. He returned to driving his car, which he had avoided since the last accident, and began actively seeking work. It was noted that his litigation still had not been settled, but he did not speak of it and seemed to have little interest when the subject was broached except that his medical expenses should be reimbursed for the interim period.

This individual had been seen by other psychiatrists who had concluded that he was suffering from a "compensation neurosis"; they predicted that when the settlement occurred everything would be well again and that he would be unsuitable for any rehabilitation program unless the litigation was settled. In fact, with some patience, it was possible to assist this man to leave the litigation in the hands of the lawyers and to get on with the business of helping himself.

Case Report

Miss O.P. This 31-year-old single woman had complained of a right shoulder pain and neck stiffness for about 5 years, since an injury at work. After a long dispute, the Workmen's Compensation Board had denied her any further entitlement, and she had made a few abortive attempts to return to work. On reviewing the file, it was of interest that 1 year prior to her injury she had been seen by a different consultant because of temporomandibular joint dysfunction which resolved spontaneously when she dropped an unsatisfactory relationship with a boyfriend.

She recalled having poor self-esteem as a child. The father was domineering, making her feel that she could not do anything right, and the mother was overpossessive. She recalled her long dependency on her parents; for example, she stayed 10 years at a job she did not like because her father had told her that she should not change jobs. It had also taken her 7½ years to extricate herself from the relationship with the boyfriend with whom she had had an unequal and unsatisfactory relationship. She was involved in a therapeutic program which included pain control classes, work stations supervised by Occupational Therapy, and general relaxation training. Progress was marginal, however, until conversations were held with the psychiatrist regarding her long fight with the Workmen's Compensation Board. She felt that she had to continue her appeals and litigation with them as a matter of principle, because, as she saw it, they had been treating her and probably many other people unfairly. The psychiatrist enabled her to recognize that maybe some of the energy she was investing in her battle had to do with her lifelong resentment at the injustice of her childhood. Whether or not she might be "morally right" she appreciated that she was wasting her life carrying on this unfruitful struggle which, at best, would eventually get her a pension that would not be worth the effort. She took the bold step of writing a letter to the Workmen's Compensation Board renouncing any further claim for the injury in question and withdrawing her application for an appeal. She then obtained a 6-week work assessment, which was sponsored by a government vocational and rehabilitation service office. During the assessment she realized that she had been interested in art all along and had never felt free to do as she liked. She now was able to successfully find a career that made use of her artistic talents and allowed her to be fully employed and totally self-sufficient.

In the above case, an important element in this individual's recovery did appear to be the cessation of litigation. The reason for the litigation was not primarily in terms of the sum of money that might have been received but rather was in terms of long-held resentments which were being displaced against the Workmen's Compensation Board. The dynamics noted in the above 2 cases give a more balanced view of the role that compensation and litigation may play in the perpetuation of chronic pain.

ILLNESS BEHAVIOR REINFORCED BY THE FAMILY

On the one hand, it must be recognized that having family support is important for a good therapeutic outcome (48). The case of J.B. mentioned in Chapter 9 illustrates this point. Psychosocial disturbance in the patient's family may also be implicated in a poor therapeutic outcome (50). For this reason, seeing family members of chronic pain patients appears to be a necessary routine practice. It is interesting that families of chronic pain patients may actually demonstrate a good deal of cohesion rather than obvious conflict, but the cohesion may involve mutual endorsement of the sick role adopted by the index member, while directing blame and anger outward against physicians, compensation boards and others. Obviously the intervention has to begin by ascertaining whether there exists some dissatisfaction within the family system. If there is some lack of stability or "homeostasis"—if the sick role has not been fully "assimilated" by the family—there may be sufficient motivation either in the patient or other family members to bring about change. Where distress is lacking, it is essential to recognize this and, instead, to work toward more limited goals. This perhaps can be done by employing a behavioral management program in conjunction with hospital admission, recognizing of course that this may deal with problem behaviors in the hospital but not necessarily show carry-over after discharge.

Case Report

Mr. Q.R. This 53-year-old man had a 16-year history of chronic low back pain and lupus erythematosus with arthritis. He was well-known to the staff of the Inpatient Rheumatic Disease Unit because of his frequent admissions and multiple dissatisfactions and complaints. He would participate poorly and complain of pain whenever he was asked to exert himself or to go for a treatment he found unpleasant. He related that he had had an injury to his back in 1964 and had asked the physicians to do an operation. They had refused at that time, saying that there was no evidence of injury. Several years later, because of an arthritic process in his hips he came to a bilateral hip replacement, which was uneventful technically and which gave him absolutely no relief. He cited these items as proof that if the physicians had operated when he first asked them to he would now be well, but because they had neglected him he was doomed to be forever disabled. He saw his admission strictly in terms of the need for pain relief and reduction of swelling in his joints. He stated that he had received many medications, and he recalled a long list of side-effects that each medication gave him. However, he accepted analgesics and codeine even though he claimed that these too were bad for him.

His support came from a small government pension. He had no workmen's compensation or entitlement because, he claimed, "they lost the file." His wife was working and he remained home all day babysitting his 3½-year-old grandson. The wife would get up in the morning and prepare all the food and things that he and the grandson would need during the day, whereas Mr. R. would do nothing on his own behalf. He claimed to enjoy the company of the grandson greatly and enjoyed telling him stories or talking with him. He reported proudly the cleverness of the little fellow, how he would set up pillows for grandfather to lie on and remind his grandfather to be sure to get his proper afternoon rest. It was evident that family members required virtually no productive activity from him. He was included by the family in social visits, but generally he had the status of an onlooker. He described his family as very understanding.

His manner of relating to the examiner reflected a note of irony, and he reported no emotional distress whatsoever. The patient saw no point in further conversations with the psychiatrist. The opinion at the time of the assessment considered the duration of his illness and the length of time away from the work force, the limitations imposed by his hip replacements and arthritis, and the family attitude as all important contributing factors to perpetuation of his problem. Nevertheless, the patient was offered admission to the Inpatient Pain Unit. At first the patient accepted but later sent an angry letter refusing any further contact. A meeting was then held between him and the ward staff, setting out the following limited management conditions. When the patient was to be admitted, the purposes for admission would be written down with an estimate of the time necessary to achieve these goals and with a statement of the amount of necessary cooperation that must be obtained from the patient to ensure a good result. Admissions were not to be prolonged beyond the agreed period or prolonged if the patient was not participating and not making best use of the program. It was recognized that the patient would probably have further admissions and that regression after discharge would be rather likely each time and, therefore, that efforts should be concentrated on minimizing the behavioral disorder and problems for staff while the patient was in the hospital.

THE MULTIPLE PATIENT FAMILY

As noted by Mohamed and Waring (Chapters 10 and 11 this volume) and as noted in other literature (43, 50, 53), it is a very frequent occurrence to find that chronic pain patients have family members who are likewise psychologically or medically impaired. It is also likely that in the case of many chronic pain patients discussion of illness may have a particularly high communication value and may be responded to rather selectively. Many times, patients will improve or fail to do so depending on whether other members of the family are becoming well or remaining ill. Conjoint family management is not only desirable but, probably, also essential.

Case Report

Mr. and Mrs. S.T. This 48-year-old man was referred because of chronic low back pain and, as usual, the spouse was invited to attend. The examiner was surprised when the patient and wife entered the room—he carrying a cane and limping and pushing his wife in a wheelchair. Eight years earlier, Mr. S.T. had had some accidents at home, followed by low back pain. Since that time he had had 4 myelograms, a chymopapain injection, a hemilaminectomy, a discectomy, 2 fusions and removal of osteophytes and had worked intermittently. He had been involved in an outpatient rehabilitation program, but since his daily activity tolerance was only 2 hr, he had not benefited.

Mrs. S.T. had developed low back pain with sciatica and right S-1 root signs over the past year, and her symptoms were getting worse. Her activity was also drastically limited and, like her husband, she showed discouragement and sadness. There were troubles also at home with 3 teenage children who had seemed to slip beyond the parents' control in recent months. Mr. and Mrs. S.T. felt at a loss as to how they could begin to set limits again.

From Mr. S.T.'s family background it was learned that his father had suffered migraines and ulcers, and his brother had likewise suffered migraines as well as having spells of "passing out" whenever he would have a pain. The psychiatrist completed the examination of both Mr. and Mrs. S.T., also having Mrs. S.T. seen by a physiatrist in the same office. The findings were discussed with both of them. They were told that his chronic pain problem would most likely benefit from an inpatient treatment program, whereas her problem was compatible with acute disc herniation without progressive neurological deficits and she would be likely to benefit from conservative physical medicine measures. While he was admitted to an inpatient program including group therapy, relaxation training, job stations, a fitness program and electrical stimulation, his wife was involved in an outpatient program including active physiotherapy and anti-inflammatory drugs. Both of them were seen in conjoint marital therapy and both improved simultaneously, with better family functioning; Mr. T. returned to work 7 weeks after initially being seen.

EPIDEMICS

Attitudes and morale are communicated from patient to patient, particularly on rehabilitation units where they have an opportunity to be together for more prolonged periods of time. This transmission of morale may have both positive and negative effects (8). On a well-functioning unit, the morale is managed well. Patients model good coping strategies for each other and learn by observation the sort of difficulties they may have to encounter and what the likely outcome will be. Expectation for a hopeful outcome is aroused by seeing others doing well and being discharged. The good morale might be taken for granted by a casual observer, but staff performance is essential in maintaining and conveying a positive affective tone. When a problem in morale occurs and the staff do not recognize it as a function of the unit atmosphere as a whole, there may be a feeling of rising irritability and discomfort on the part of staff, who may make referrals, asking for patients to be transferred or for the psychiatrist to visit.

Case Report

An emergency psychiatric consultation was requested regarding a 53-year-old man who had been admitted with osteoarthritis of both knees and who had been unable to work for 2 years. He had a longer history of low back pain. This patient was in great distress, calling out at night, crying or shouting at the nurses, refusing to get out of bed for scheduled activities, and constantly asking for analgesia. When staff members tried to reason with him, he threw his food across the room at them. At interview he was noted to be greatly apprehensive, lying in bed and complaining bitterly, crying and stating that he feared a catastrophic progress of his back pain and arthritis. He had lain in bed at home for virtually 7 months before this admission. The arthritis of the knees had been occasioned by falls at work and knee surgery, and eventually he had been dismissed from his work because he could not climb—he felt this to be grossly unjust but saw no possibility of returning to an employable status. He had skills at the master electrician level and was obviously an intelligent individual. During his younger years he had survived internment as a prisoner of war, had come as an immigrant to Canada, had been an important individual in a veterans' association and had been successful in his work. The examiner had the impression that the patient idealized his premorbid functioning and that he certainly catastrophised his current state. It appeared that the disruptions on the ward had not been present at the time of admission but had arisen recently as the patient had suddenly begun to feel very hopeless about the admission and about his future, felt that nobody was listening to him and thought that something serious that he did not understand was going wrong.

Down the hallway, shouts could be heard from another man obviously in distress, and on inquiring at the nursing station the psychiatrist was told that there were in fact 2 other patients who were giving them a great deal of difficulty: a man with ankylosing spondylitis who was bedridden and a woman with arthritis and complications of steroid medication. The other man was examined and found to be an elderly gentleman who probably always had been difficult to get along with and was now showing unmistakable signs of dementia. After being admitted to the hospital, the patient had become progressively more disoriented in a strange environment and had begun to shout, defecate, and be resistive. The female patient was also interviewed. She had been in hospital several months and after initially doing fairly well had suddenly run into some serious complications from her steroids. This had left her feeling unwell and alarmed for her safety. She had responded to the setback by spells of panic, weeping, crying out at night, withdrawing to her room and feeling hopeless.

Although these patients were in different rooms and had not actually spoken with each other, they were all within earshot of each other and were being attended by the same group of nursing staff. Furthermore, the problems had erupted at approximately the same time, although 2 of the 3 patients had been in hospital for a longer period prior to the disturbance. The staff were feeling a good deal of frustration and were asking for these patients to be transferred to the pain program or to a psychiatric ward. The elderly man responded to a program of eliminating drugs which impaired the sensorium and providing regular orientation and having family members visit. The 2 other patients were involved in a group which was operating for chronic pain patients on a different ward. They formed warm attachments to other chronic pain patients with whom they could identify and feel understood, and the behavior problems abated.

IMMIGRANTS WHO HAVE BEEN INJURED

There are discussions in the literature dealing with individual, personal, family, and cultural differences in pain expression (41, 66, 70). Whether cultural differences actually affect therapeutic outcome in most cases is difficult to establish. First generation immigrants are more heavily represented among the group of laborers who are at higher risk for industrial injury and, for that reason, would be seen in clinics or consultations for workmen's compensation (30). Apart from the question of whether high risk exists, it is apparent that, at times, immigrants are for various reasons at a disadvantage after being injured. Some of the reasons for being disadvantaged relate to problems that they particularly might face, whereas other factors may relate to the setting in which the injury occurs.

People who immigrate are apt to be highly motivated people who have a great personal need to improve their status in life and improve the family future. They may have small social support and little capital and recognize the need to succeed while they are still young and healthy. Injury for them would be catastrophic in its significance since they have fewer financial and social options for their survival other than a return to health. People who migrate seeking work may also be a special breed of individuals who personally place a high value on getting ahead and succeeding. Failure for them may be more feared. It may make matters worse if things were going poorly at the time of injury so that the injury became "the final straw"—in such a case, chronic pain may become a rationale for failure. The workers compensation system into which a laborer may be precipitated can offer a disincentive for a return to health because it provides enough income for a minimum survival, but it does not provide enough to ward off anxiety. There may be a fear that attempts to return to work may fail but will be punished nevertheless by removal of a pension. There may be cultural differences in how much illness complaints are tolerated within a family or extended family. This might be further influenced by language and social isolation that a family may feel in a new setting. In this way, a sick member and a family might be less influenced by the broader social context of attitudes and there may be a tendency to take a "paranoid position" in feeling let down by the new country.

The medical system also may reflect some societal differences. If illness complaints are thought to be more "deviant" in North American society than in a country of origin, the patient may feel subtle messages that he is not being believed. If in the country of origin medical professionals are given a more authoritarian role, treatment by their current physicians, who may not be able to speak the patient's language, may be mistrusted. There may be a tendency for North American physicians to attribute problems to psychological causes, and to someone who knows of psychiatry only in an institutional role this may seem to be tantamount to an accusation of madness.

Evidently, the factors cited above would equally apply to a native-born individual without family supports, to a family that moves from one location to another in this country, and to someone with limited education who does not understand what is happening to him in the medical system. The issue then may be that the problem of the injured immigrant is only more apparent because certain problems of chronic illness and disability are particularly highlighted. The matter, nevertheless, bears consideration because it is reasonable to believe that the most important issue is the availability of a social support system on which to fall back when injury or other difficulty occurs. This may heighten the need for the family as a whole to receive support at the same time that the index patient is being seen.

Case Report

Mr. U.V. This 45-year-old Italian man suffered low back pain and was first seen in company with his wife. A few years before, he had managed to develop a family bakery business and things were going fairly well. Fire broke out and Mr. V. reached for the extinguisher which came loose from the wall and threw him backwards so that he injured his back. By the time the firefighters came, the business was essentially destroyed and, unfortunately, was underinsured. From that time he suffered severe low back pain and received a partial pension from the Workmen's Compensation Board. There was a marked loss of ability to function at home and several attempts at rehabilitation were unfruitful. In one work placement in a bakery he would have sudden falls without warning or explanation, and he was unable to carry on. He believed that his only salvation would be in total alleviation of his pain. On examination it was noted that he was using a cane, wearing a brace, and sometimes walking better than at other times. There was a positive bow-string sign, a reduced ankle jerk, and relative numbness in S1 distribution in one leg, and there was tenderness in the low back and in the posterior musculature of the neck. He was involved in the Inpatient Pain Treatment Unit, and transcutaneous nerve stimulation was tried but was accompanied by exacerbation of the pain. Antidepressants produced nightmares and agitation. His attitude in group therapy consistently reflected a feeling of hopelessness that things could be any better. As he saw it, he had come to Canada to make a better life for his family. Some of his children were already of university age, and to provide for them as he felt he ought would require him not only to be well but also to work overtime. If he did not have the strength to do more than an average day's work, as he saw it, his future was bleak. Often he did not participate in assigned work stations or physiotherapy, and he had frequent falls without warning. It was noted that sometimes he would walk with a cane in one hand and sometimes in the other, but he could not be persuaded to discard the cane. When told that he was not making satisfactory progress after several weeks, he accepted the comment with resignation as if he had expected this verdict all along.

In this case, it seemed that the attitude this individual bore toward his disability was closely linked to his situation and personality rather than to linguistic or cultural differences. This case is probably fairly representative of many patients who are unable to accept and benefit from a rehabilitation program.

Conclusion

Psychiatrists consulting to rehabilitation clinics and wards have the advantage of training in medical skills and concepts as well as expertise in psychological intervention. This blend of skills and concepts is particularly valuable for rehabilitation patients and chronic pain patients for whom both the medical and the adjustment and psychological variables must be considered. Management of chronic pain and disability can occur directly through the skills of the psychiatrist in contact with the patient as well as through facilitating the development of programs by the treatment team and other nonpsychiatric professionals. It is appropriate for psychiatrists to accept leadership in some areas of rehabilitation of patients with chronic pain.

REFERENCES

1. BARBER, T. X. Measuring hypnotic-like suggestibility with and without hypnotic induction. *Psychol. Rep. 16:* 809–844, 1965.
2. BECK, A. T. *Cognitive Therapy and the Emotional Disorders.* International University Press, New York, 1976.
3. BEECHER, H. K. Relationship of significance of wound to pain experienced. *J.A.M.A. 161:* 1609–1613, 1956.
4. BISHOP, D. S. (Ed.) *Behavioral Problems and the Disabled.* Williams & Wilkins, Baltimore, 1980.
5. BLOCK, A. R., KREMER, E., AND GAYLOR, M. Behavioral treatment of chronic pain: Variables affecting treatment efficacy. *Pain 8:* 367–375, 1980.
6. BLOCK, A. R., KREMER, E. F., AND GAYLOR, M. Behavioral treatment of chronic pain: The spouse as a discriminative cue for pain behavior. *Pain 9:* 243–252, 1980.
7. CAIRNS, D., THOMAS, L., MOONEY, V., AND PACE, J. B. A comprehensive treatment approach to chronic low back pain. *Pain 2:* 301–308, 1976.
8. CRAIG, K. D. Social modeling influences on pain. In *The Psychology of Pain*, edited by R.A. Sternbach. Raven Press, New York, 1978, pp. 73–104.
9. CRAIG, K. D., AND PRKACHIN, K. M. Social modeling influences on sensory decision theory and psychophysiological indexes of pain. *J. Pers. Soc. Psychol. 36:* 805–815, 1978.
10. DELAPLAINE, R., IFABUMUYI, O. I., MERSKEY, H., AND ZARFAS, J. Significance of pain in psychiatric hospital patients. *Pain 4:* 361–366, 1978.
11. DEVINE, R., AND MERSKEY, H. The description of pain in psychiatric and general medical patients. *J. Psychosom. Res. 9:* 311–316, 1965.
12. ENGEL, G. L. Psychogenic pain and the pain-prone patient. *Am. J. Med. 26:* 899–918, 1959.
13. FINNESON, B. E. Modulating effect of secondary gain on the low back pain syndrome. In *Advances in Pain Research and Therapy, Vol 1*, edited by J. J. Bonica, and D. Albe-Fessard. Raven Press, New York, 1976, pp. 949–952.
14. FORDYCE, W. E. Behavioral concepts in chronic pain and illness. In *The Behavioral Management of Anxiety, Depression and Pain*, edited by P. O. Davidson. Brunner/Mazel, New York, 1976, pp. 147–188.
15. FORDYCE, W. E., FOWLER, R. S., LEHMANN, J. F., DeLATEUR, B. J., SAND, P. L., AND TRIESCHMANN, R. B. Operant conditioning in the treatment of chronic pain. *Arch. Phys. Med. Rehabil. 54:* 399–408, 1973.
16. FRANK, J. D. Common features of psychotherapy. *Australia N.Z. J. Psychiatry 6:* 34–40, 1972.
17. GREENHOOT, J. H., AND STERNBACH, R. A. Conjoint treatment of chronic pain. In *Advances in Neurology, Vol. 4, Pain*, edited by J. J. Bonica. Raven Press, New York, 1974, pp. 595–603.
18. GRZESIAK, R. C. Chronic pain: A psychobehavioral perspective. In *Behavioral Psychology in Rehabilitation Medicine; Clinical Applications*, edited by L. P. Ince. Williams & Wilkins, Baltimore, 1980, pp. 248–300.
19. HENDREN, R. L., AND KRUPP, N. E. Reintegrating psychiatry into pain-management programs. *Psychosomatics 20:* 229–232, 1979.

20. HERMAN, E., AND BAPTISTE, S. Pain control: Mastery through group experience. *Pain 10:* 79–86, 1981.
21. HILGARD, E. R. The alleviation of pain by hypnosis. *Pain 1:* 213–231, 1975.
22. HOHL, M. Soft-tissue injuries of the neck in automobile accidents: Factors influencing prognosis. *J. Bone Joint Surg. 56-A:* 1675–1682, 1974.
23. KERR, F. W. L. Craniofacial neuralgias. In *Advances in Pain Research and Therapy: Vol 3*, edited by J. J. Bonica, J. C. Liebeskind, and D. G. Albe-Fessard. Raven Press, New York, 1979, pp. 283–295.
24. KHATAMI, M., AND RUSH, A. J. A pilot study of the treatment of outpatients with chronic pain: Symptom control, stimulus control, and social system intervention. *Pain 5:* 163–172, 1978.
25. KLEE, G. D., OZELIS, S., GREENBERG, I., AND GALLANT, L. J. Pain and other somatic complaints in a psychiatric clinic. *Md. St. Med. J. 8:* 188–191, 1959.
26. KOSTERLITZ, H. W., AND TERENIUS, L. Y. (Eds.) *Pain and Society*. Verlag Chemie, Weinheim, 1980, pp. 93–382.
27. LARGE, R. G. The psychiatrist and the chronic pain patient: 172 anecdotes. *Pain 9:* 253–263, 1980.
28. LASCELLES, R. G. Atypical facial pain and depression. *Br. J. Psychiatry 112:* 651–659, 1966.
29. LIEBMAN, R., HONIG, P., AND BERGER, H. An integrated treatment program for psychogenic pain. *Fam. Process 15:* 397–405, 1976.
30. LINDSAY, J. The injured workman: Do cultural influences affect his rehabilitation? *Can. J. Occup. Ther. 38:* 15–19, 1971.
31. MARBACH, J. J., AND LIPTON, J. A. Aspects of illness behavior in patients with facial pain. *J. Am. Dent. Assoc. 96:* 630–638, 1978.
32. MARUTA, T., SWANSON, D. W., AND SWENSON, W. M. Chronic pain: Which patients may a pain management program help? *Pain 7:* 321–329, 1979.
33. MEICHENBAUM, D., AND TURK, D. The cognitive behavioral management of anxiety, anger and pain. In *The Behavioral Management of Anxiety, Depression and Pain*, edited by P. O. Davidson. Brunner/Mazel, New York, 1976, pp. 1–34.
34. MERSKEY, H. Psychiatric aspects of the control of pain. In *Advances in Pain Research and Therapy, Vol I*, edited by J. J. Bonica, and D. Albe-Fessard, Raven Press, New York, 1976, pp. 711–716.
35. MERSKEY, H. Psychiatric management of patients with chronic pain. In *Persistent Pain*, edited by S. Lipton. Academic Press, London, 1977, pp. 113–128.
36. MERSKEY, H., ET AL. Pain terms: A list with definitions and notes on usage. *Pain 6:* 249–252, 1979.
37. MERSKEY, H., ET AL. The principles of pain management: Group report. In *Pain and Society*, edited by H. W. Kosterlitz, and L. Y. Terenius. Verlag Chemie, Weinheim, 1980, pp. 483–500.
38. MERSKEY, H., AND BOYD, D. Emotional adjustment and chronic pain. *Pain 5:* 173–178, 1978.
39. MERSKEY, H., AND EVANS, P. R. Variations in pain complaint threshold in psychiatric and neurological patients with pain. *Pain 1:* 73–79, 1975.
40. MERSKEY, H., AND HESTER, R. A. The treatment of chronic pain with psychotropic drugs. *Postgrad. Med. J. 48:* 594–598, 1972.
41. MERSKEY, H., AND SPEAR, F. G. *Pain: Psychological and Psychiatric Aspects*. Ballière, Tindall & Cassell, London, 1967.
42. MITCHELL, K. R., AND MITCHELL, D. M. Migraine: An exploratory treatment application of programmed behaviour therapy techniques. *J. Psychosom. Res. 15:* 137–157, 1971.
43. MOHAMED, S. N., WEISZ, G. M., AND WARING, E. M. The relationship of chronic pain to depression, marital adjustment, and family dynamics. *Pain 5:* 285–292, 1978.
44. MOLDOFSKY, H., SCARISBRICK, P., ENGLAND, R., AND SMYTHE, H. Musculoskeletal symp-

toms and non-REM sleep disturbance in patients with "fibrositis syndrome" and healthy subjects. *Psychosom. Med. 37:* 341–351, 1975.

45. MOLDOFSKY, H., AND WARSH, J. J. Plasma tryptophan and musculoskeletal pain in non-articular rheumatism. *Pain 5:* 65–71, 1978.

46. NEWMAN, R. I., SERES, J. L., YOSPE, L. P., AND GARLINGTON, B. Multidisciplinary treatment of chronic pain: Long-term follow-up of low-back pain patients. *Pain 4:* 283–292, 1978.

47. ORNE, M. T. Mechanisms of hypnotic pain control. In *Advances in Pain Research and Treatment Vol I*, edited by J. J. Bonica, and D. Albe-Fessard. Raven Press, New York, 1976, pp. 717–726.

48. PAINTER, J. R., SERES, J. L., AND NEWMAN, R. I. Assessing benefits of the pain center: Why some patients regress. *Pain 8:* 101–113, 1980.

49. PILOWSKY, I. Abnormal illness behavior and sociocultural aspects of pain. In *Pain and Society*, edited by H. W. Kosterlitz and L. Y. Terenius. Verlag Chemie, Weinheim, 1980, pp. 445–460.

50. ROBERTS, A. H., AND REINHARDT, L. The behavioral management of chronic pain: Long-term follow-up with comparison groups. *Pain 8:* 151–162, 1980.

51. ROMANO, M. D. Staff problems in rehabilitation. In *Behavioral Problems and the Disabled*, edited by D. S. Bishop. Williams & Wilkins, Baltimore, 1980, pp. 365–377.

52. SCHACHTER, S., AND SINGER, J. Cognitive, social, and physiological determinants of emotional state. *Psychol. Rev. 69:* 379–399, 1962.

53. SHANFIELD, S. B., HEIMAN, E. M., COPE, N., AND JONES, J. R. Pain and the marital relationship: Psychiatric distress. *Pain 7:* 343–351, 1979.

54. SICUTERI, F. Headache as the most common disease of the antinociceptive system: Analogies with morphine abstinence. In *Advance in Pain Research and Therapy, Vol 3*, edited by J. J. Bonica, J. C. Liebeskind, and D. G. Albe-Fessard. Raven Press, New York, 1979, pp. 359–365.

55. SPEAR, F. G. Pain in psychiatric patients. *J. Psychosom. Res. 11:* 187–193, 1967.

56. STEGER, H. G., FOX, C. D., AND FEINBERG, S. D. Behavioral evaluation and management of chronic pain. In *Behavioral Problems and the Disabled*, edited by D. S. Bishop. Williams & Wilkins, Baltimore, 1980, pp. 302–336.

57. STEGER, J. C., AND BROCKWAY, J. A. Management of chronic pain in the disabled. In *Behavioral Problems and the Disabled*, edited by D. S. Bishop. Williams & Wilkins, Baltimore, 1980, pp. 272–301.

58. STEINMULLER, R. The use and abuse of psychiatry in dealing with pain patients. *Psychiatr. Q. 51:* 184–188, 1979.

59. STENGEL, E. *Pain and the Psychiatrist*. Medical Press, New York, 1960, pp. 28–30, 243.

60. SWANSON, D. W., MARUTA, T., AND SWENSON, W. M. Results of behavior modification in the treatment of chronic pain. *Psychosom. Med. 41:* 55–61, 1979.

61. SZASZ, T. S. The nature of pain. *Arch. Neurol. Psychiatry 74:* 174–181, 1955.

62. TAUB, A. Relief of postherpetic neuralgia with psychotropic drugs. *J. Neurosurg. 39:* 235–239, 1973.

63. TITCHENER, J. L., AND ROSS, W. D. Acute or chronic stress as determinants of behavior, character, and neurosis. In *American Handbook of Psychiatry*, Ed. 2, edited by S. Arieti. Basic Books, New York, 1974, pp. 39–60.

64. TUNKS, E., AND MERSKEY, H. Psychiatric treatment in chronic pain. In *Behavioral Problems and the Disabled*, edited by D. S. Bishop. Williams & Wilkins, Baltimore, 1980, pp. 238–271.

65. WARD, N. G., BLOOM, V. L., AND FRIEDEL, R. O. The effectiveness of tricyclic antidepressants in the treatment of coexisting pain and depression. *Pain 7:* 331–341, 1979.

66. WEISENBERG, M. Pain and pain control. *Psychol. Bull. 84:* 1008–1044, 1977.

67. WEISENBERG, M. The regulation of pain. *Ann. N.Y. Acad. Sci. 340:* 102–114, 1980.

68. WILSON, R. R., AND ARONOFF, G. M. The therapeutic community in the treatment of chronic pain. *J. Chron. Dis. 32:* 477–481, 1979.
69. WOODFORDE, J. M., AND MERSKEY, H. Some relationships between subjective measures of pain. *J. Psychosom. Res. 16:* 173–178, 1972.
70. ZBOROWSKI, M. *People in Pain.* Jossey-Bass, San Francisco, 1969.
71. ZEIG, J. K. (Ed.) *A Teaching Seminar With Milton H. Erickson.* Brunner/Mazel, New York, 1980.

14

Synthesis and Future Directions

ELDON TUNKS, M.D.
RANJAN ROY, Adv. Dip. S.W.
ANTHONY BELLISSIMO, Ph.D.

Arriving at this part of the book, the reader has encountered a variety of concepts, several viewpoints, a number of procedures for intervention and hopefully some thought-provoking issues. The various chapters have dealt with concepts and observations ranging from the medical to the sociological and theoretical frameworks covering the sociocultural, overt (operant) behavioral, covert (cognitive) behavioral, and psychophysiological perspectives. The ever-increasing diversification of both models and intervention strategies points to the conclusion that the "puzzle" of chronic pain is yet to be resolved. Faced with a multiplicity of concepts and theoretical systems, how does one achieve a coherent "psychosocial" synthesis that has application to the "rehabilitation" of the chronic pain patient?

This chapter takes up the challenge of integration, in a preliminary way, by analyzing some of the themes and issues raised by the various chapters in the book. The intent of such analysis is to move toward the following future objectives:

1. To provide conceptual unity to the understanding of chronic pain and, eventually, of chronic disability in general. This conceptual unity is visualized not as an idiosyncratic one but as one that builds on and is more or less parallel to other important conceptual frameworks in general use (e.g., ego-psychology and object relations theory, general systems theory, and language and communication theory). It must have sufficient integration and stability to be portable beyond chronic pain (e.g., other "psychosomatic" disorders).

2. To provide a basis for confidence in clinical approaches to chronic pain. Realizing that to date we have failed to solve the problem of chronic pain, more active links between the clinical and research

literature are needed in order to work toward providing "proven" intervention systems. A framework is needed that encourages continued productive development of future therapeutic approaches.

It is evident that the above are long-term objectives and are not likely to be achieved in the immediate future.

Major Themes of the Book

Although the writers in this book have addressed various aspects of chronic pain, the primary emphasis has been on intervention. (Five of the chapters in the body of the book focus on various modes of intervention.) In addition to intervention, another emphasis is pervasive throughout the book. This is the exploration of psychological and sociological concepts for their relevance to the understanding of chronic pain. These attempts using psychosocial viewpoints to examine and understand chronic pain are at their best when they complement biomedical perspectives. The blending of the psychosocial and the biomedical perspectives stems, in part, from the awareness that, even when the chronic pain is associated with organic damage, psychosocial variables play an important part in maintaining and/or aggravating the problem.

Several more specific themes can be identified in this book. These themes will be listed here and then discussed:

1. *Psychological fields or dimensions.* Several axes can be followed through the book. These can be categorized as 1) overt (social-environmental, operant-behavioral) and 2) covert (cognitive-behavioral, psychophysiological).

2. *Definition of pain problem.* A number of developments can be followed in this area. These include the movement from the concept of pain simply as a symptom to the concept of pain as the object of consideration in its own right: the shift from the speculative, introspective and post hoc to the pragmatic, experiential and immediate.

3. *The contextual or ecological focus.* This theme emphasizes the phenomenon of chronic pain as it occurs in its natural context. The development of this theme reaches the conclusion that chronic pain is primarily the manifestation of a dysfunctional system, and the system becomes the unit of treatment.

4. *Adaptational focus.* The theme here is shift of control and responsibility to "self-management" and "problem solving."

5. *Medical treatment-education polarity.* In the area of chronic pain, this theme follows the conceptual development which shifts the focus from "cure" to "relief" and from patient passivity to the educated action of the consumer.

6. *An analysis of the nature of intervention.* Considering the large array of treatment options, why do different interventions work, and on what systems do they act?

PSYCHOSOCIAL FIELDS OR DIMENSIONS

It is not new to point out the fallacy of the "body-mind dichotomy," and there is little resistance to its criticism. Engel (3) and Wolff and Langley (17) note that dualistic approaches to disease are undesirable. The real problem is in finding coherent alternatives, since the currency of our technical language is bound up in these older ideas. Even medical specialties are divided along "body-mind" lines, so that, in practice, patients are categorized and streamed. Szasz (16) was attempting to address this when he advanced the position that pain is simultaneously a sensation (private) and also a communication. Merskey and Spear (11) attempted to circumvent the dualism issue by proposing a "monistic" definition of pain. This solution is reflected in the definition of pain endorsed by the International Association for the Study of Pain (10). "Pain is an unpleasant sensory and emotional experience which we associate with tissue damage and describe in terms of tissue damage." Sternbach (15) took an analogous position, that pain is a unitary experience that is modulated by several ever-present factors (essentially biological, psychological and social). A transcultural study by Fabrega and Manning (4) examined Ladino views of disease and pain in the Chiapas Highlands of Mexico. They noted that dualistic notions of pain did not even appear in the terminology that natives used to describe distress. They were more prone simply to identify an unpleasant sensation and, if pressed for explanation, would begin to attribute this to matters of constitution, impressionability, and circumstance, without apparent bias toward relevance of any of these factors.

Exactly how one chooses the conceptual axes on which to base models is dependent on the issue under study. Melzack and Wall (9) in elaborating the "gate theory" of pain proposed three axes: 1) sensory-discriminative, 2) cognitive-evaluative and 3) affective-motivational. All were seen to interact in the pain event. The integrative and multidimensional focus continues to appear in recent reviews, with the assertion that treatment may be more effective when interventions are targeted at more than one subsystem (Cameron, Chapter 7) (14). All of the chapters in this book, in fact, underline this attitude. Cameron divides the psychosocial field into environmental, psychophysiological, cognitive and behavioral. Yet, he notes that there is no real integration yet in discussion of various psychosocial subsystems (and maybe there never should be).

One domain in which intervention must be made when "abnormal illness behavior" (Chapter 8) presents, is the public one. Even with individual psychotherapy, as noted by Bellissimo and Tunks (Chapter 9), the sufferer meets with a representative of society. More obviously, operant treatment methods (reviewed in Chapter 7) apply a special set of societal expectations and sanctions to elicit change. Sociologically, these may be effective programs because they suppress the absolution that society normally grants its sick members, emphasizing instead the duty to get well.

In Chapters 4, 5 and 6, attention is given to the social dimension with respect to the sick role and its ramifications in the special cases of the injured worker and women in pain. Tunks and Roy (Chapter 5) discuss the social dimension as comprising several overlapping fields, including societal, occupational, familial, and illness roles in addition to the "personal role" or "script."

Family dimension and roles also have much to do with the illness role being perpetuated or not, and a natural unit of treatment is the family (Chapters 10 and 11). Waring notes that even in the particular strategy of family therapy, there are a number of psychosocial subsystems that might receive attention. The operant family therapy model gives much attention to the field of cues and reinforcers. The structural model uses systems and communication theory parallel to an ego-psychology formulation of family members. The cognitive family therapy taps the private field of covert behavior at the same time that communication and problem solving function are facilitated. To this list of options should be added the McMaster model, essentially a systems model, which considers systems within systems and breaks functioning down into affective vs. instrumental, problem solving, communication, roles, affective responsiveness, affective involvement, and behavior control (2).

In short, an alternative to dualistic conceptualization involves two elements, a multidimensional model which includes psychological and social dimensions and a definition of pain which does not confine itself to implying a unitary "cause" (e.g., "psychogenic" or "organic" pain) but names the distress itself.

DEFINITION OF THE PAIN PROBLEM

A major stimulus to redefining pain as a problem in itself rather than the symptom of something underlying has been the clinical problem of individuals who complain of pain but whose apparent pathology does not explain the problem. Violon (Chapter 3) articulately describes the need felt in such a case for medical legitimizing, and her solution, compatible with the empathic stance of the doctor, is to define and treat it as a disease (algopathia). If it is medical legitimizing, it is based on presentation of a multi-factorial consideration of the problem. Giving it a name should not distract us from that. It is a broader conceptualization than "abnormal illness behavior." To give it a name, to satisfy the "principle of Rumpelstiltskin" (5), probably facilitates the doctor-patient engagement, but not without problems. Is it really better than simply reassuring the patient that chronic pain like this is not uncommon and that it is believable? On the other hand, the process described by Violon does fairly represent the strategy employed by the majority of pain clinics, and most pain doctors do "give it a name"—"fibrositis," "panalgesic syndrome," chronic "soft tissue injury," etc. It might also be argued that after a while the "disease focus" becomes counterproductive (13). If inherent in a label there is nothing to suggest a mechanism that can be understood and reversed, the label may provoke anxiety and mystification instead of being reassuring.

Definition is also needed regarding whether chronic pain is a medical or rehabilitational or, even more generally, a social problem (as in the case of alcoholism being handled by AA). Gallagher and Wrobel (Chapter 4) make the point that medicine has, in a way, "colonized" the problem of chronic pain, in much the same way that, for example, childbirth has become a medical issue. Maybe such colonization is not necessary or even desirable. (Alternatives will be discussed below.) All of this bears, however, on the matter of definition of chronic pain in the broadest sense. Is it a medical issue alone, or is it social or divided, or does medicine stand in by proxy for the rest of society? The definition is important because it defines the resources, tasks and tools.

In almost every chapter of the book, mention is made of the need to demonstrate acceptance of the reality and affliction of the pain. Does such definition impose a hidden condition that the patient may not be responsible to solve his own problem? (Gallagher and Wrobel, Chapter 4, talk about exemptions.) What about the sanctions imposed by operant conditioning programs? Surely implicit in them is the fact that the chronic pain problem remains at least in part the responsibility of the sufferer.

Agreeing that there is a necessity to accept the patient's complaint, such messages have to be communicated in a way that avoids the absurdity of telling the patient that he does not feel what he claims to feel. Merskey (Chapter 2) helps with the definition of pain he proposes. This definition moves the understanding of pain from the somatic to the experiential domain.

The need for definition does not rest just with pain doctors. There is the problem of communication by other health professionals about pain patients, to avoid the problem of speaking in what seems to be an esoteric way about pain and not run the risk of losing too much information or encouraging overgeneralizations. Baptiste and Herman (Chapter 12) discuss the process of introducing patients to group therapy. A feature is "indoctrination," in which a conceptual model is taught in lay language with the purpose of setting a base for reevaluating the pain problem. The same point is made by Pilowsky and Bassett in terms of the "negotiation stage of therapy" (Chapter 8). In doing so, a "language" is taught which unites the client and therapist (5). As Gallagher and Wrobel point out, the redefinition of the pain problem must eventually lead to reconceptualizing of both the patient's and the therapist's roles, and the process leads to creation of new sociomedical institutions.

CONTEXTUAL OR ECOLOGICAL FOCUS

The contextual focus has been a point of major emphasis throughout this book. It would probably be correct to say that what pain clinics bring uniquely to the modern scene is precisely this ecological and social focus as well as methods taken from psychosocial services. Several contexts are examined. Violon and Gallagher and Wrobel discuss the confrontation between the sick role, which is accepted in traditional medicine, and the chronic sick role, which arouses suspicions and problems and which calls for a medically nontraditional approach. Pilowsky and Spence (13) have talked about "abnormal illness behavior" as characterizing some chronic pain patients. In these discussions, it is pointed out that part of the chronic pain patient's problem is his "legitimacy" and that that is understood in terms of the sociomedical context.

Another context is that discussed by Crook (Chapter 6) the complaint of a woman in pain in the context of long-standing popular conceptions and normal roles (in the sense of general). Does the idea that "it is part of the woman's normal life-cycle to be ill and in pain" still influence our thinking? What about the fact that social benefit systems and habilitation systems seem less ready to deal with women on the same basis as with other injured? What is "return to normal" for a woman with chronic pain?

The pain complaint as a function of disrupted working role and the consequent multiple role change is detailed by Tunks and Roy (Chapter 5). It becomes debatable whether this is chronic pain treatment any more or some form of politics.

The family is probably the most important unit of intervention in rehabilitation (and treatment of chronic pain). Taking the specific example of cognitive family therapy, covert behavior is examined in context of interpersonal dysfunction. In structural family therapy, the identified complaint is examined in context of family and family-therapist function. Social groups can also be reconstituted as with forming a therapy group. Here the effects of modeling and interpersonal persuasion are mobilized on the premise that gains will be generalized to other social contexts. As Cameron discusses (Chapter 7) and Baptiste and Herman describe (Chapter 12), new adaptive learning may be best in a controlled therapeutic situation where more than one psychosocial subsystem can be accessed.

Gallagher and Wrobel note that ethnic issues are somewhat ignored. Although ethnic differences in response to pain have been researched (18), findings have not shed much light on what should be done in any particular case. Pain clinics are flooded with injured migrant workers who seem to have a worse prognosis than do other pain patients. The reasons for this can probably be found in culturally different notions of acceptable illness behavior, unfamiliarity with current cultural milieu and responses, enhanced uncertainty due to language barriers, economic vulnerability and family isolation which can lead to paranoid attitudes.

ADAPTATION

Gallagher and Wrobel, Cameron and Baptiste and Herman all observe that pain patients can alter their experience of pain by various methods or strategies (Chapters 4, 7, and 12). Presumably the same potential for suffering still exists. Adaptive changes can also be traced in family and occupational settings. When change is desired, change in the whole environment may have to be induced. It is interesting to recall Cameron's discussion of biofeedback training. Evidently, psychophysiological effects are not nearly as specific as one would expect. One wonders about the specificity of many other favorite pain clinic treatments, whether they work instead by giving the necessary rationale: a sense of mastery and an impetus for self-management and problem solving.

A pillar in management of chronic pain is insight oriented, or supportive psychotherapy, as described by Pilowsky and Bassett (Chapter 8), but Bellissimo and Tunks (Chapter 9) observe that pain patients are not, in general, good candidates for psychotherapy in the traditional sense, and Baptiste and Herman (Chapter 12) warn against mixing pain patients with general psychiatric patients in a therapeutic setting. Therapies are vehicles for therapeutic persuasion and education, inducing rehabilitative change, and several chapters emphasized the role of taught coping strategies. Their methods and language probably have to be derived from the problems and experience of pain patients to be effective (the same way that psychoanalytic theory and method arose from people who were psychologically minded and identified themselves as distressed in this way).

MEDICAL TREATMENT—EDUCATION POLARITY

It would seem from reading Violon's and Cameron's chapters that if the treatment of chronic pain is medicine it is a modified form of it. Gallagher and Wrobel note that there is a shift from absolute emphasis on care to relief. The vehicle of education and rehabilitation is used. Analogies can be drawn between self help programs for the public and the "behavioral medicine" trend for chronic pain patients. The same point has been made by Sanders (14). On the one hand, complex psychosocial rehabilitation strategies have been rather uniquely mounted in pain clinics. On the other hand, medicine may be relatively deskilled and disadvantaged by "colonizing" a problem for which it lacks special resources, training or even credibility (Chapters 4 and 9). For now, pain clinics will probably go on adopting resources and skills they need. The use of the popular press and media for advocating fitness, diets, and health awareness, the jogging and bicycling movements, and the introduction of "educational" formats into the health scene all seem to reflect a shift from medical monopoly to public ownership of problems such as "stress control," life-style and "pain control."

THE NATURE OF INTERVENTION

Cameron (Chapter 7) correctly observes that, in certain technologies such as biofeedback, therapeutic application and instrumental refinement is well ahead of supportive research. (The same could be said, for example, about transcutaneous electrical nerve stimulation.) In the example of biofeedback, Andrasik and Holroyd (1) showed that therapeutic benefits were linked to conditioned physiological change, but much less specifically than would be imagined. Similar questions had been raised years ago regarding the active ingredients of psychotherapy in comparison, for example, to those of dynamic and behavioral therapies (8). Critical investigation of both new and old intervention technologies is needed to sort out effective from less effective methods and specific from nonspecific factors if confidence is to be built in therapeutic practice.

The question above can be further expanded to, "Why is any effective treatment effective?" The beginnings of a model to address this question might be seen in the work of Frank and his colleagues (6).

The essential elements of therapeutic persuasion include:

1. Sufferer and healer, culturally defined, are in therapeutic contact.
2. Rationale, in which healer is expert, binds healer and sufferer together—"Rumpelstiltskin is named."
3. "Rationale" provides explanation for problem and proposes routes for solution.
4. Focus is agreed upon for therapeutic endeavor.
5. Rituals based on "rationale" offer opportunities for mastery: the sufferer is motivated, expects positive outcome, holds the therapist in esteem and is actively engaged in the ritual.
6. Rituals offer opportunity for further arousal of emotion and motivation.
7. Application is made to the context of original problem.

These elements might alternatively be called the "nonspecific" factors in therapy. This is almost an anthropological model with broad scope, applicable to everything from psychoanalysis to shamanism or the fringe psychotherapies or biofeedback. Undoubtedly, such a model is useful because of its generalizability, but, by the same token, it lacks specific detail that would enable someone to select the most appropriate intervention for a particular case. In other words, it suggests why an intervention might or might not be successful in a certain instance but does not provide a basis for mounting the intervention itself; for this, a more specific and less generalized model is required (such as psychodynamic, operant, information processing, or psychophysiological).

The conceptual model that is chosen as a basis for intervention also defines the unit of concern, whether this be some psychophysiological process, some thought that is linked to an action, or perhaps a social interaction. For example, in family psychotherapy the focus is not on the complaint nor on the index patient but rather is on the "family process"; the therapist, as a participant in the system, influences it so that it might shift to a new equilibrium.

Individual and family treatment options may lie fairly within medical (psychiatric) practice, but some group "education" programs (Chapter 12) constitute something closer to social intervention. It is also interesting to note that such programs have also tended to spawn self-help or "alumni" groups (7, 12).

As long as representatives of the health professions adopt chronic pain treatment, with its biological, psychological and social dimensions, as an area of expertise, interdisciplinary activity and multiple conceptual models will be necessary. Here, we come full circle to the motive for compiling this book. What beginning can be made in this without becoming too esoteric, complex, or reductionistic? Will this provide a forum for learning/teaching skills for concepts that will make a "pain therapist"?

Peering into the Crystal Ball

Peering into the crystal ball, we first see reflected the panorama of what is already around us: a new definition, refined conceptual models and some innovative applications.

A much more acceptable set of definitions of pain terms, that endorsed by the International Association for the Study of Pain, is currently available (10). To clarify and agree on the meaning intended by such terms as "pain," "hyperpathia," "hyperalgesia," and "hyperesthesia" are essential both for communication and for conceptual clarity.

As reviewed in this book, a large array of conceptual models is available for discussing pain—many of these models involve psychosocial concern. It must be remembered that concepts are tools for understanding and action and, like tools, may be more suited for some tasks than for others. Some concepts are very broad, suited, for example, for describing the effective ingredients in a variety of interventions (6). Some concepts such as the gate theory of pain lack general relevance but may serve to describe how emotional events might modify a painful event. Some other concepts such as ego-psychology models might suggest particular avenues that may help a patient alter his emotional state that is bound up with his pain. Different conceptual levels of analysis are needed, depending on the task. The operating anesthetist needs his biomedical model. The social worker equally requires his family systems model.

Looking a bit into the future, there may develop a renewed awareness of the importance of the "philosophy of medicine," and pain clinics will need philosophers to facilitate interdisciplinary interaction if pain treatment is to remain coherent and integrated.

We do not need a crystal ball to see that increasing longevity and the exponential rise in cost of medical technology are forcing the public to appreciate that we cannot have everything that is scientifically possible to do. This awareness may have something to do with the popular swell of interest in jogging, fitness, diets, and life-style management. As the gap between the affordable and the technologically possible widens, the public will be further impelled to again assume ownership of life-style, stress control, and chronic pain and disability. The way may be led by innovative but effective sociomedical systems such as the "pain control classes" and self-help groups. Furthermore, we may be able to envision a new social structure in which medicine may choose to play less of a part—a "life/ health management profession."

REFERENCES

1. ANDRASIK, F., AND HOLROYD, K. A. A test of specific and non-specific effects in the biofeedback treatment of tension headache. *J. Consult. Clin. Psychol.*, *48:* 575–586, 1980.
2. BISHOP, D. S., AND EPSTEIN, N. B. Family problems and disability. In *Behavioural Problems and the Disabled*, edited by D. S. Bishop. Williams & Wilkins, Baltimore, 1980, pp. 337–364.
3. ENGEL, G. L. Psychogenic pain and the pain-prone patient. *Am. J. Med.*, *26:* 899–918, 1959.
4. FABREGA, H., AND MANNING, P. K. An integrated theory of disease: Ladino-Mestizo views of disease in the Chiapas Highlands. *Psychosom. Med.*, *35:* 223–239, 1973.
5. FRANK, J. D. Common features of psychotherapy. *Austr. N. Z. J. Psychiatry 6:* 34–40, 1972.
6. FRANK, J. D., HOEHN-SARIC, R., IMBER, S. D., LIBERMAN, B. L., AND STONE, A. R. *Effective Ingredients of Successful Psychotherapy.* Brunner/Mazel, New York, 1978.
7. HERMAN, E. Pain control: A group approach. Paper presented at International Association for Study of Pain, Second World Congress, Montreal, August, 1978.
8. MARMOR, J. Common operational factors in diverse approaches to behaviour change. In *What Makes Behaviour Change Possible*, edited by M. A. Burton. Brunner/Mazel, New York, 1976.
9. MELZACK, R., AND WALL, P. D. Pain mechanisms: A new theory. *Science 150:* 971–979, 1965.
10. MERSKEY, H., ET AL. Pain terms: A list with definitions and notes on usage. Recommended by the IASP Subcommittee on Taxonomy. *Pain 6:* 249–252, 1979.
11. MERSKEY, H., AND SPEAR, F. G. *Pain: Psychological and Psychiatric Aspects.* Ballière, Tindall, and Cassell, London, 1967.
12. NEWMAN, R. I., SERES, J. L., YOSPE, L. P., AND GARLINGTON, B. Multidisciplinary treatment of chronic pain: Long-term follow-up of low back pain patients. *Pain 4:* 283–292, 1978.
13. PILOWSKY, I., AND SPENCE, N. D. Illness behaviour syndromes associated with intractable pain. *Pain 2:* 61–71, 1976.
14. SANDERS, S. H. Behavioural assessment and treatment of clinical pain: Appraisal of current status. In *Progress in Behaviour Modifications, Vol. 8*, edited by M. Hersen, R. M. Eisler, and P. M. Miller. Academic Press, New York, 1979, pp 249–291.
15. STERNBACH, R. A. *Pain: A Psychophysiological Analysis.* Academic Press, New York, 1968.
16. SZASZ, T. S. The nature of pain. *Arch. Neurol. Psychiatry 74:* 174–181, 1955.
17. WOLFF, B., AND LANGLEY, S. Cultural factors and the response to pain: A review. *Am. Anthrop. 70:* 494–501, 1968.
18. ZBOROWSKI, M. *People in Pain.* Jossey-Bass, San Francisco, 1969.

Index